What Readers Have Said About

Living Binge-Free's
Message of Hope

. . . *an inspiring example of the new generation of self-help books . . . the principles are universal in application . . . . growth takes guts and that, as much as the sterling advice, is what this book is about.*
> David Alan Ramsdale, MEDITATION Magazine

A very, very honest, personal and comprehensive approach to dealing with disordered eating . . . . helpful to anyone struggling with those issues themselves.
> Marcia G. Hutchinson, Ed.D. Author, Transforming Body Image

No other book on this topic has taken its readers so far down into the darkest depths of the hell of the disease. . . through the painful rollercoaster ride of the recovery process . . . into the freedom and ecstasy of a binge-free life. It is an empowering book of encouragement and hope. . . .
> Julie J., recovering from multiple compulsive disorders

. . . *concise, articulate and organized. . . . offers a positive, workable approach to change and recovery . . . . an excellent resource and a very encouraging guide . . .*
> Changing Woman Magazine

I was emotionally moved at times, hopeful at the practical steps offered and very very excited to realize that bulimia is not an incurable disease!
> Grace Elizabeth Bell, Denver

. . . *penetrating . . . highly recommended: [going] beyond the usual methods of defining illness to suggest concrete paths for recovery.*
> Midwest Book Review

When I read it, I couldn't wait to get back to it every time I had to stop. . . . Thank you very much. I have a feeling of excitement and hope from its words.
> Recovering bulimic

. . . *moves the reader beyond the mechanics of recovery and into the living process of spiritual transformation . . . a deeply personal account of one woman's search for spiritual fulfillment through the dark passage of despair. . . . Its message is authentic.*
> Carol Riddle, New Age WOMAN

This book is testimony to the fact that compulsive eating is curable . . . an inspiration for women to challenge our culture's destructive obsession with being thin.

Kim Lampson Reiff, Ph.D., Psychologist and Recovered Bulimic Anorexic

. . . excellent. . .

International Psychologist

If you want a book that covers both the personal experience of a compulsive overeater and recovery solutions that work, this book is it. I enthusiastically recommend this book . . .

Brett Valette, Ph.D. Author, A Parent's Guide to Eating Disorders

. . . an informative account . . . clear, easy to read. . . .

Journal of Nutrition Education

I find this work to be most intriguing, informative and well written. It should be an asset to anyone desiring to find the tools necessary to deal with this horrendous condition.

Bill B. Author,, Compulsive Overeater and Maintenance for Compulsive Overeaters

I found your book to be very helpful — much inspiration. I have newfound hope to overcome this demon.

A Reader in Minnesota

. . . a practical, readable nine-step guide.

Good Spirit

This is a heart-told story of a woman's victory over compulsive eating. Shattered by the multi-billion dollar diet industry, Jane Latimer shares, step-by-step, how she rediscovered her body's inner wisdom. I recommend that all my clients read this extremely insightful book.

Mary Taylor Montgomery, M.S., R.D., Nutrition Consultant

Jane
Evans
Latimer

LIVING

BINGE-

FREE

A Personal Guide to Victory Over Compulsive Eating

LivingQuest Publishing Company
Denver, Colorado

Library of Congress Cataloging in Publication Data.

Latimer, Jane Evans, 1948-
    Living Binge-Free: A Personal Guide to Victory Over Compulsive
Eating
    Bibliography: p. 137
    Includes index.
    ISBN 0-882109-00-7
    1. Bulimia -- Treatment. 2. Compulsive eating --Treatment.
I. Title.
RC552.B84L37 1988
615.85'2--dc19   88-15899
                                                            CIP

© 1988 by Jane E. Latimer

Cover Design by Bob Schram/Bookends
Cover Photograph by Tom Irwin

Published by LivingQuest Publishing Company
                Box 101412
                Denver CO 80250
                (303) 692-9162

Printed in the United States of America
10 9 8 7 6 5 4

The Self lies quietly within. When we are still, we can hear it speak. As it manifests outward, we feel a deepening of inner power. From our Self comes our ability to know, to heal. Your Self knows right now what it is you need to do to recover.

This is the story of my journey, and my journey alone. To try to imitate it would be a great mistake. As you read, listen to your Self silently. At certain times you may hear a stirring -- this will be your cue to act.

This book is dedicated to:

my parents, for all they have given me,
my husband, Gene, who taught me how to nurture myself,
my children, Jesse and Cory, who taught me how to nurture others,
all children, that they may grow up with self-love, and indeed,
all people willing to change, that we may come to know our true Selves.

Acknowledgements

I am most grateful to the many people who contributed their time, support and feedback toward the making of this book. A very special thanks to you all: my husband, Gene, for putting in hundreds of hours listening, reading, re-reading, editing and reassuring me when my doubts prevailed; my friends Julie, Linda and Mary Jane for help with my earliest manuscript; Barbara Cohn for reviewing the manuscript in detail and giving me much needed advice and support; the many professionals who took time to read it and give me their invaluable feedback — Bill B, Marcia Hutchinson, Vivian Meehan, Mary Montgomery, Kim Lampson Reiff, Esther Rome, Jacquelyn Small and Brett Valette; the bulimics and overeaters who read the early versions and offered badly needed advice; Kim Mooney and John Kadlecek, my editors, for excellent work; Bob Schram, my graphic designer, for managing to capture the vision inside my head; Johann Robbins and Tom Irwin for jobs well done; Barbara Cohn, Sue Evans, Bob and Lee Evans for generous financial support; and last, but certainly not least, Meme Latimer, Laurie Frain and the moms in my babysitting co-op, who freed me from the demands of motherhood long enough to make this project a reality.

There would never have been a book, however, if I had not learned to live binge-free myself. For all of you who played your role in my recovery, may the Universe return manyfold all the love and help you gave me: Dr. Crannendonk for helping me open the door to my rage; Rosemary Feitis (and, indirectly, Ida Rolf) for helping to set the stage for my spiritual awakening; Dr. Ira Progoff for giving me tools to find my own inner wisdom; and especially those who led me through my spiritual infancy, counseling and guiding me through my darkest night until I learned to see the Light within — Ralph, Crystal, Penny, Wyndee, Jan, Bruce, Rebekah, Lois, Jon, Dorothy, Toby — and, of course, Russell, who showed so many of us the way.

CONTENTS

Introduction

More than just the story of my life and recovery, this book is a set of guidelines leading out of the twisted maze of obsessive/compulsive eating. It is not an exact map by any means, but a description of processes by which you, directed by your own inner wisdom, can learn to navigate your course out of this trap into the rest of life that exists beyond food and eating.

I began overeating when I was eleven years old. Until I was twenty-four I binged mainly at night, starved myself throughout the day and exercised rigorously to maintain a relatively normal weight. My binges started after supper and lasted until bedtime when I would fall asleep, painfully stuffed, only to awaken again in the middle of the night and resume bingeing. The mornings were times of despair and resolve never to do it again. My days were filled with calorie-counting — often carrying a full schedule in school and dance classes on only two hard boiled eggs and a cup of plain yogurt.

When I was twenty-four, after a long, difficult relationship that finally broke off painfully, I became bulimic. My binges increased in quantity ten-fold and increased in frequency to three to five times a day. Always, without fail, these binges were terminated by self-induced vomiting. This behavior lasted seven years until my full recovery at age thirty-one.

My recovery began when I first realized that I had an illness. In the beginning, a small part of me wanted help, but most of me didn't. The first step of my recovery was to find and keep in touch with the part that wanted to be healthy. Most of the time I was unaware it was there, but through the years it got larger and stronger until it became strong enough to actually override the compulsive drive.

At the time of this writing I am thirty-nine years old, happily married, with two sons. I have not binged in eight years. I have been asked if I ever binge, even just a little. My answer is always "No."

At one time I used food as a defense to protect me from looking at and confronting the parts of myself that I didn't want to see. I had to find the strength to take a look. I didn't want to at first and only did so a little at a time. I took only what I was willing and able to handle, and that was why the recovery was slow — but it was steady. The larger my capacity for self-confrontation grew, the more I was able to change and the healthier my eating patterns became.

Self-discovery is a journey inward. At the center lies the Self. For those of us with an addiction the movement inward is painful, but it is precisely our willingness to go through that pain that enables us to bring about permanent emotional and behavioral changes.

1

Living Binge-Free is the story of my recovery; but more than that, it is the story of my willingness to peel off unwanted layers — obsession with food, emotional trauma, self-destructive behavior — and find within myself a true place of being that is uniquely mine to own.

I've attempted to present an outline of the stages of this very special journey. This was a particularly challenging task, as those stages are mere memory, no longer a part of my present life. The section on food was an incredibly difficult section to write because food has ceased being an issue for me.

Please keep in mind that while I was actually working on freeing myself, I stumbled along, confused and unknowing. It is only in retrospect that I've been able to put the pieces together, to analyze the actions and attitudes responsible for my complete recovery in hopes they will open a pathway, inspire an action and act as a guide for you.

Although I had very little therapy (at the time I was recovering there weren't any "eating disorder clinics" or therapists specializing in eating disorders), I did have help. I did not go it completely alone. I saw counselors, and I became a member of a large support group. Although much of the work I did was on my own, the guidance I received was irreplaceable. I would suggest that while it is important to learn to listen to your own inner voice, it is also important to know when to ask for help. Professional help can be invaluable. If I were struggling with this problem today, I would without question find a well qualified therapist. There are many excellent programs in existence today. Not to utilize them would be wasteful.

My personal reflections and journal writings are scattered throughout. I hope that they will touch your heart and provide inspiration and deeper insight into the process of change. For me, change is the miracle of life. Without it there is no hope, no reason for living.

PART ONE

YOU CAN CHANGE

Rachel said some very good things to me today. Learn to love the subtle experiences. They are times of slower and more imperceptible movement, but without them the large changes could not be made.

My body, me, some part of me is saying "No, I do not want to grow and work on growth. Go away, growth." Growth is a beautiful name. It comes in disguises from the inside but appears to be from the outside. Growth is always with us. Growth is my home. Sometimes I want to leave home and run away from myself.

Growth is the internal Self expanding as it inherently should and will. It takes on varied forms and directions infinitely.

– April 23 1974

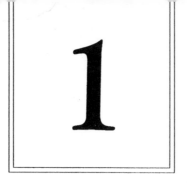

The Spiritual Journey – to Selfhood

The True Self

The addict has a special journey, a journey to Self. The true Self, the strongest, most powerful and most solid part of us, can only be reached, in the beginning, by moving through pain. The pain happens when we begin to penetrate the surface of our small existence, through the conditioned overlays that have served to protect us from an environment that often seems hostile and threatening.

In order to find that Self again, we must be willing to strip ourselves of the conditioned overlays, go back to childhood and recontact that vulnerable and naked place. Then we can begin to rebuild the house in which we live, a house that can become as our Self always wished it to be. Otherwise we run the risk of staying stuck in the place of despair. Once eating behaviors are stripped away and the temporary high of superficial thinness is attained, we begin to wonder what this is all about. Is this all there is?

A life of thinness and healthy eating cannot sustain our deeper needs as individuals. We realize after the initial thrill, we are left living by rote, just as unthinking in our day-to-day life as we once were in our need to overeat. Herein lies the danger of setback. To sustain our recovery, we must look deeper. We must find a way to stay in contact, on an ongoing basis, with the needs of our Self. We must learn to listen and to act on the wishes of that Self. This is what I mean by the spiritual journey — it is the journey to Selfhood.

Power — "The ability to do, act or produce."
Webster's New World Dictionary, Second College Edition

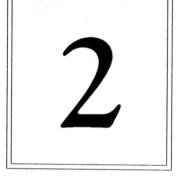

On Personal Power

Freeing Your Energy

When I was a child, power seemed to exist only outside of myself. My parents had power — so did my teachers, the police, government officials, even the bullies at school. I certainly didn't.

Most of us tend to think of power as being the ability to influence or control others; we hardly think of power as being something simple like an "ability to do, act or produce." When we speak of personal power, however, we are speaking of just that.

Power is applied or focused energy. Energy is the fuel for doing, acting or producing. If our energy is blocked, our capacity for action will be handicapped. If our energy is abundant, we will be able to act effectively.

Energy can be increased in many ways. The healthier we are, the more energy we will have. The more in touch with Self we are, the more we act on our true or best behalf, supporting ourselves and our actions with the free-flowing energy of the universe.

People who suffer from eating disorders will never know their potential for personal power until they begin releasing the energy that is trapped in that behavior. Those behaviors act much like a dam. The river's source of abundant energy and force comes from within, from Self. It flows outward until it is blocked by the dam of repressed feelings, low self-esteem, lack of motivation, fear of intimacy, attitudes, perceptions and habitual eating patterns conditioned by others and society. As these old behavior patterns are broken up, a river of energy will be released.

I found my own personal power by unplugging that dam. I began feeling my feelings, loving myself, acting on my desires, sharing myself with others and expressing myself unashamedly.

I feel a personal mission to help women transform the conditioning that shapes our attitudes towards ourselves, food and our bodies. To live powerfully is to have the energy to manifest our true self potential as human beings. We cannot do this if we are caught in a daily battle with our own bodies — the number of calories we consume, the shape of our legs, buttocks and breasts. Take a look at how much energy you spend counting calories, overeating, starving, vomiting, etc. If you were able to reroute that energy into achieving personal, financial and career goals, you would have an enormous reserve upon which to act. Your life could be amazingly exciting and fulfilling. Think about it!

What a magnificent tree

I sit on my front steps, my heart aching. I look at a tree that sits in my front yard. I sketch its outline with my eyes. As I do, I move into the center of that tree. I feel its life, its glory. I never saw that tree before. It's beautiful with its cracked branches, not a perfect tree, not the kind of tree you'd notice in passing and say, "What a magnificent tree." Just a very plain tree and yet as I look, it opens itself to me and reveals its soul to me and says "I am a glorious tree, a being of grandeur. Thank you for taking the time to see me for who I am."

I become aware of my eyes, how they are a vehicle through which life can communicate. If I use my eyes to look, life enters through them. Most of the time I do not use my eyes in this way. I use them as most of us do. They see to help me go through the motions of living – do my chores, direct my movements, accomplish my daily tasks – not a small feat by any means, but a task that if done day in and day out without reflection results in feelings of meaninglessness.

But when I stop to use my eyes the way God meant them to be used, I see life the way God meant me to see life, through my soul. I contact the inner life of things and, thus doing, I see meaning and feel meaningful.

Before I wrote these words I was in despair. I sat looking at my front yard, but I never saw that tree. My mind was racing — "I hate where we live, when will we move, I pine for my dream house, acres of mountain land. Will we ever be able to make it happen?" My heart ached. My mind raced. I was forlorn, already feeling like a failure.

It was at this point many times before, many years before, that I would have gone to the refrigerator, stuffed myself and fallen asleep only to awaken feeling guilty and ugly. But the worst sin of all was that I missed the moments of bright living, sharing and feeling that could have happened. If I had let myself move through the despair, to the other side, if I had let life guide me in its wisdom and direct me as to the action I was to take, I could have changed many years of my life.

Today I was guided to get my notebook and search in writing for the meaning of my despair. In the process I felt the grief move my mind to question the nature that surrounded me. My eyes moved to that tree, caressed that tree, touched it. It touched back with its inner being and lifted the despair that was in my heart.

In all life there is suffering. Why do we expect there not to be? Let's not run away from despair, afraid to feel it. Only when we allow ourselves to feel pain are we also able to feel the magnificence of life and to know the ultimate meaning and purpose behind our otherwise shallow existence.

I believe compulsive eating is a cry for help, a cry of despair. I believe that behind the facade of bingeing and dieting is a very lost being, a sad being, a being unable to find a Self, a being that lives an empty and disconnected life.

Through the shallowness of this existence we pass ourselves by. It's tragic. Yet, just as I chose to look deeply at that tree, we can learn to look deeply at ourselves and, when we do, find a secret Self — powerful and glorious — even in all of its imperfection.

This book, in a sense, is about that imperfect tree. It is written for you, an imperfect being, and comes out of the experience of my own imperfect self.

That tree stands in my front yard and it says, "I am who I am. I have power and beauty because I am who I am with my broken branches. I know no other way. I am proud. I stand with dignity."

— November 11, 1986

I wake up. It is the middle of the night. It is dark and the house is quiet. Depressed, and in a cold sweat, I touch my thighs and stomach. They feel too big. I feel sick. I did it again last night. I hate myself. Why can't I stop?

Quietly I slip out of bed in the dark. Moving slowly, careful not to wake my sister, careful not to make a sound, I grope my way down the hall, using my hands to guide the way. I know this path by heart. I've done this many times before.

I hear a sound in the bathroom. One of my parents is awake. I wait, my heart beating. I must be sure they don't suspect I'm here. The toilet flushes and then the house is quiet again. I wait. Everything is quiet.

Cautiously I approach the kitchen and quietly close the door. Now I can relax. The light from the refrigerator illuminates the room. My hand reaches for the freezer. I pop a couple of pieces of frozen bread into the toaster. My fingers grab a glob of vanilla ice cream. When the toast is ready I spread it with cream cheese and pop two more frozen pieces of bread into the toaster. Grabbing a handful of Fig Newtons, still munching on the toast, some part of me realizes what I'm doing. The tears begin to run down my cheeks. Why can't I stop? My head hurts... mouth still full of cookies... I'm aware of my hand reaching for the leftover meatloaf. I grab some meat... can't take the time to cut it... can't stop... toast, cheese, cookies, peanut butter... stomach hurts... pain. I'm sobbing now. Please dear God, why can't I stop? My stomach is about to burst, and my eyes are wet with tears. My heart explodes with pain; my lungs are tight; I have a hard time breathing. Grabbing a handful of graham crackers, I make my way painfully, slowly, back to my bed.

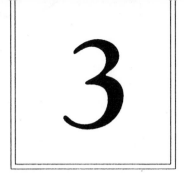

MY STORY

Who I was. My Recovery. Living Binge-Free.

Although I started eating compulsively when I was eleven years old, it was during high school that I became obsessed with my body. Every waking moment was uncomfortable and stressful. My body was changing, and I was ashamed. I wanted it to remain the body of a little girl — no soft curves, no roundness, no thighs, no breasts, no hips. I was growing into a woman, and I was frightened. I did not want to grow older, but the changes my body was going through would not let me forget. That was why I turned against it. To me, it was the enemy, pushing me into places unknown, places I was frightened of, places I refused to go.

Everything that was wrong was blamed on it. "If only I could be a normal eater, if only I could be thin and beautiful, then I would be happy." If only...if only...if only.... I never looked beyond the surface.

The images projected on the pages of *Vogue* and *Mademoiselle* became my reality. I strove to be like them. My attraction to and infatuation with the magazine models was a source of endless grief. No matter how hard I tried, I couldn't make myself look like them — my breasts, hips and thighs were too big, and my hair too frizzy. In my dreams I believed I could be Cinderella, but when I glanced at myself in the mirror, all I saw was the ugly duckling.

So, I separated myself from others — avoided the kids at school, stayed away from boys and did not go on dates. I became disinterested in the things that other girls my age seemed to fuss over — boys, clothes, parties. I needed to feel I was better than them because I felt so worthless deep inside.

Then I started dance classes. It was something I was good at. I was talented and encouraged to work at it. I loved the attention. I knew I had a special talent, and people liked to watch me dance. Maybe they were jealous or envious. This gave me pleasure too.

I protected my loneliness with the belief I would be another Nureyev one day. I covered my despair and fear of sex with my obsession for perfection. Dancing made me feel special. It also helped protect me from the real and painful issues of my life — loneliness, despair, anger and fear. With food, I stuffed and starved my body. With dancing I tried to push, pull, stretch and bend it into the shape I wanted it to be — shapeless.

My body would not listen. I looked in the mirror and I saw not the lithe, long look of a Balanchine form, nor the slender, chic look of a *Mademoiselle* model. I saw instead, the full breasts and spreading thighs of a woman.

Disgusted, I refused to eat. I was a success every day until dinner, when I would surrender to that overpowering craving for food. From the moment I took that first bite, I would be unable to stop.

I was first introduced to drugs in high school by our family doctor who prescribed diet pills to help me control my weight. They controlled my hunger and boosted my energy level.

During my first two years of college I experimented heavily with hallucinogenic drugs. I alternated the "acid" trips and marijuana food orgies with twenty-four hour spells of "black beauty" amphetamine highs, during which time I ate nothing. This kept my weight within a ten pound range.

When I graduated, I had to face the harsh realities of making my own way in the world. I wanted to be an artist, so I rented a run-down loft in New York City. The place was old and filthy. The wood was rotting; electrical wires hung from the ceiling. There was no shower or kitchen, but there were two johns. So, with the help of a friend, I managed to turn one of the bathrooms into a shower. My grandparents gave me an old refrigerator, and I bought a hot plate to cook on. This served as my kitchen for the following seven years.

On the floor beneath me, a Greek family ran a pretzel factory. I awoke every morning to the sounds of chattering Greek and the smell of hot burning coals. A large two-ton garbage bin sat outside into which stale and soggy pretzels were thrown away each evening. These pretzels later became the mainstay of my midnight bulimic binges.

I began dating a man who, as I look back on it now, was both an alcoholic and a compulsive eater. Steve hid his illness behind a wild and glamorous front. He had charisma and money. He was a much sought-after, young American artist.

I fell in love with him, I thought. What I really fell in love with was his power, independence and wealth. Part of me "knew" I couldn't make it on my own, that I had to have someone to depend on. Another part wanted to be like him — powerful, successful, rich and independent.

Our evenings were spent at bars. When drinking, he never ate. This meant he often went two to three days without food. We'd drink at night, come home and watch the late movies on TV, sleep most of the day and start out again the next night. After a few evenings of this, bored and wiped out, we'd stay home and rest in front of the television set. He'd give me $50 to go buy some of everything from the nearby deli or Chinese takeout. I ate until I was numb with stomach pain and emotional helplessness. He consumed quantities of food which, up until then, were previously unknown to me. His frequent jaunts to the toilet suggested to me he was vomiting his food, but I never knew for sure.

I hated everything we did together, but I needed him to love me. I needed to believe I could be loved by a man as powerful and successful as him.

As our relationship degenerated I began to feel I had failed miserably as a woman. I desperately needed to believe it would right itself again and refused to let our relationship go. I couldn't face the emptiness that would threaten to consume me if I did let him go. In truth, I was afraid to face the fact that I could not provide for myself, that I felt I had failed as an artist, and that I was filled with emotions I didn't understand.

When I finally admitted that he and I were through, my bingeing escalated.

After we split up, the emptiness was unbearable, and I turned to food for consolation. My suspicions that Steve vomited suggested an alternative to getting fat: I could binge all I want, yet remain thin, pretty and desirable. Food became an all-consuming, uncontrollable obsession.

At one time, the size of my binges were limited by how much my stomach could physically hold; now there was no limit. I would gorge until I could hold no more, then stick my finger down my throat, bend over the toilet bowl and vomit until every morsel had been eliminated and there was room to gorge some more.

From the time Steve and I split up until my recovery seven years later, I was incapable, for the most part, of controlling my eating behavior. And yet, for the first three years I didn't even know there was anything wrong. I thought I had found an ingenious way of controlling my weight, that my binges were merely extensions of an already established eating pattern begun in high school, nothing to be seriously concerned about.

I don't know how I could have had such misperceptions about my behavior. My life was ruled by my obsession. I worked nights at a job where I had free time, flexibility and no co-workers. I would come to work with two big quarts of cole slaw, wash the mayonnaise off in the ladies' room (to save the

13

calories), eat them during the first few hours and then would search the wastebaskets for left-over lunches that had been thrown away by daytime employees.

I would leave work at midnight and take a bus that let me off a couple of blocks from an all-night deli. I'd buy a loaf of bread, cream cheese, a box of cookies, a package of cheese and a quart of ice cream. When I got home I'd head straight for the bathroom, sit down on the floor and eat until I couldn't hold anymore. Then I'd stick my finger down my throat, throw up, and finish what was left over. Dehydrated, eyes and neck in pain, I'd get into bed and fall asleep feeling miserable about myself and what I'd done. Some nights I'd wake up, creep downstairs and grab eight to ten dirty, soggy pretzels from the two-ton garbage bin outside my door. Staring blindly at the wall, I'd chew hard and fast. I'd be sure to wash them down with milk or water, as they were very hard to vomit and even then I had to convulsively gag them up and out.

I made friends with a little man who owned a seedy coffee shop around the corner from my loft. He began preparing to open for breakfast around 2:00 a.m. and would sell me day-old pastries at half-price in the wee hours of the morning.

When I visited my friends in Vermont I'd sneak their food, then make my way in the dark outside, dig a hole and vomit in the woods. The next day, I'd go to the little general store and try to replace what I had eaten.

The vomiting hurt my eyes; they felt as if they were being pulled out of their sockets. The muscles in my neck were tight and hard. My body became uncomfortably dehydrated, and my energy was drained. I was not in a condition to work or do anything.

Most often after a binge I would fall asleep. As the years progressed and after I started actively trying to recover, I made sure I did something that would help me feel better. I'd swim, jog, sit in a sauna or get some form of bodywork or massage. All of those things helped to regenerate the normal energy flow within my body.

When I first realized I needed serious help with food, a friend of mine introduced me to Overeaters Anonymous (OA). Overeaters Anonymous is a twelve-step recovery program for compulsive eaters. It believes that overeating is a three-fold illness — physical, emotional and spiritual. Its emphasis is on the twelve-step emotional and spiritual program that has been so successful in similar programs like Alcoholics Anonymous. Although there were things about the program I did not agree with, it was my only hope for sanity, and I stuck with it.

When I first walked into an OA meeting, I knew I had found a resting place. There was hope and inspiration in the voices of its members. People shared openly and honestly from their hearts. They offered me "sanity one day at a time." I was made to feel at home by the love I felt emanating from the room. I knew I would heed their words, "keep coming back" — and I did, for the next three years.

During this time I became familiar with many new concepts, such as "Higher Power," and "abstinence." A member of OA who had been working the program longer than I became my guide or "sponsor." He helped me handle my food, and explained the twelve steps to me. I was told to write my next day's food-plan down every evening and "call it in" to my sponsor. My plan consisted of weighed and measured mealtime portions with nothing in between. Being abstinent simply meant adhering to this plan.* As I became abstinent and began working the twelve-step program, I achieved many days and weeks of "sanity," or peace of mind. I was free to experience life in a whole new way. This was a time of great emotional release. I had found a group of people who I felt understood me, and I was able to trust others for the first time in my life, allowing myself to feel and express some of the deep pain and hurt I'd kept bottled up for so many years. I became aware of my loneliness and tried to reach out to others. This was very difficult to do, however, and I continued sporadically to use food to fill the emptiness.

OA was my lifeline for approximately three years, and I attended meetings three to five times a week. At times I believed there was truly a "God" present in those rooms. I learned to hug, to cry, to trust, to be real. I learned how to become aware of my own character faults without judgment and about surrendering to a Higher Power.

However, it was not until I had my own private spiritual awakening (described later) that I came to experience Higher Power. It was, ironically, my own personal belief and commitment to following this Higher Power that finally led me away from the OA program.

Around this time, I also attended my first Intensive Journal Workshop with Dr. Ira Progoff. Dr. Progoff has developed a unique method of journal writing. It is an instrument that, if used correctly, can help a person identify the underlying direction and potential of his or her life. The Intensive Journal process is a series of progressive exercises which helps a person reconnect with the inner content and continuity of his life. As I worked with this process I

---

* At the time of this writing (at least ten years after my experience with OA), OA no longer places a lot of emphasis on food-plans and food sponsors. In fact, in some areas of the country, it may prove difficult to find a food sponsor.

began to understand the circumstances of my life from a larger perspective; events and relationships that had heretofore appeared random took on inner meaning. I had never before been given such an effective means of looking within for guidance. Its therapeutic value lay in its method of allowing me to draw upon my own inherent resources for healing. It was this power of deep contact that gave me the strength and courage to proceed forward on a predominantly self-directed path towards health.

A few months later I heard about a bodywork technique called Rolfing. The purpose of Rolfing is to put the body into alignment with gravity. This rebalancing is accomplished through ten hour-long manipulation sessions that loosen the connective tissue that surrounds the muscle. Often, emotions that have been trapped in the structures of the body are released and, in this respect, it has therapeutic value as well.

On the way home after my second session I felt an energy, a Presence, so powerful it changed the way I was to perceive my world from that time forward. As I had been raised without religious training and therefore had few spiritual preconceptions, this experience became a major turning point in my life. From that moment on, my healing was to take place on a spiritual as well as an emotional and physical level.

Inside of a month or so I found a spiritual training program that was to guide me (along with my journal work) for the next twelve years. In that program, I was taught how to tap into and direct the enormous reserve of pure energy that lies within, and I learned how to find the blocks within myself which obstructed that energy flow. It was this daily contact with my inner Self that gave me the strength and power to change. When I started working with life-energy for self-directed healing and growth, I knew I had found the way that was going to help me achieve complete recovery.

To me this meant I would one day eat like a normal eater. I would not have to weigh and measure my food or call my food plan into a sponsor every day. It meant that I could eat one scoop of ice cream or a couple of cookies and be content. I wouldn't need to eat unless I was hungry and would stop when I was full. It meant I would have power over my life and food and could survive without attending OA meetings. That is what I aimed for, and OA did not support that. So, as I got stronger within myself and started making outside friends, I let go of the OA support group.

When it became possible for me, after several years of working on my emotional well-being, to have an intimate relationship with a man without clutchiness, jealousy, fear and hate, I met the man who was to become my husband. It was the first long-term relationship that I had had in my life that was born of friendship and mutual respect.

When I met Gene, I was still bingeing and vomiting. At first I tried to hide this from him, but something deep inside said, "No." And so it was, that from the day he let me use his toilet to vomit in, he became my major means of support. He listened to my bingeing stories, consoled me and talked to me about what I was feeling. He pointed out my faults and weaknesses in a kind way, and because I knew he cared for me, I was able to accept and learn from his criticisms.

When I decided to take the plunge and change the way I ate, I first had to make a commitment to stop vomiting. I fought my fear of fat with love. For the first time in my life I began to feel okay about my body.

I then had to stop bingeing altogether. I eliminated all foods that could trigger a binge and simplified my life — took a stressless job, watched television, bathed, jogged, got bodywork, saw a few close friends, wrote in my journal and talked to Gene a lot.

Together, we made it through. Slowly I was able to take back "forbidden" foods. I was careful to watch how my body reacted, and at the first sign of a craving I would eliminate them again. As the year progressed, I realized I could eat just about anything. Thrilled by my ability to eat "normally," I went through a "junk food" stage. Today, I stay away from sugars and refined flours for health reasons and because I now prefer more natural foods, not because I'm afraid of bingeing.

For me, recovery is knowing I need never use food again to solve my problems. It has been eight years since I binged, eight years since I've even thought of bingeing. I no longer experience cravings, and I no longer need to run away from myself. I've learned how to meet life head-on. I know how to feel, how to cope with conflict and stress. I am comfortable with my body and accept my weight for what it is. I still have faults, am far from perfect, but I enjoy the challenge of growing.

Most of all, I have learned to look within for fulfillment. The joy I feel for living is the joy I get from Self unfolding. Recovery is a way of living that is committed to journeying inward. In a sense, we all must recover from our addiction to externals. That is what life is about — the journey back to our Source.

I've always had a secret desire to quilt but felt it was something only grandmothers did, so I didn't pursue it. Then one day I met a young quilter and signed up for private lessons. I fell madly in love with the process of painting my own fabric, designing the quilt pattern and sewing. It blossomed not into an "old lady's" hobby, but a true artistic endeavor that filled me with so much excitement I hated to go to sleep at night and couldn't wait to continue the next morning.

Who had time to eat?

What Are You Recovering To?

What Do You Want to Be? Ask.

We are so used to thinking of recovery in terms of "leaving behind" the state of illness, that few of us think of recovery in terms of what it is we are recovering to. Where are you going with your recovery? What are you recovering *to*?

It is not enough to wish to be free from an eating disorder. It is imperative you think about what it is you want from your life. If you say you want freedom from illness, you again are only speaking in terms of what you don't want, not what you want.

The recovery process will be easier once you begin to define who it is you wish to be as a recovered person. Ask yourself, "What am I recovering *to*?" Then proceed to answer this in affirmative statements. Your recovery will be your own; no one will be able to duplicate it.

What I recovered to:
Self-acceptance — I stopped beating myself up over every mistake I made.
Imperfection — I no longer was controlled by my "ideal" and accepted that it is an imperfect world.
Nurturance — I gave myself what I needed. I slept when I was tired, ate when I was hungry, loved when I felt empty. I enjoyed my solitude when I needed to be alone and I shared with others when I needed to express myself.
Intimacy and vulnerability — I allowed others into my life. I trusted.
I found alternative means of relieving stress — sharing, exercising, meditation, bodywork, saunas, jacuzzis and walks.
I found alternative means of coping — sharing problems, dialoguing, journal writing, communicating with Self, dreamwork, reflecting and meditating.

I enjoy life. These are some activities that give me pleasure: painting fabric, quilting, cooking, hiking, movies, talking, shopping, swimming, yoga and stretching.

Most of all, I enjoy making my dreams and goals a reality.

EXERCISE

This exercise will help you get in touch with what you want out of recovery.

With pen and paper in hand, sit in a comfortable chair. Relax, be still and quiet. Close your eyes. Breathe deeply and continue to do so until you are very relaxed. While in this deep and quiet space, feel into a typical day of your present life. What activities occupy your time? What thoughts? What feelings? What is the general pace of your life? The overall feeling?

Now get specific. Ask yourself the following questions and jot the answers down. It is very important to remain in a passive, serene state of mind while you do this. Do not lose your connection with this deep place.

How much time do I spend on enjoyable activities?

What are these activities?

What feelings occupy most of my time?

What thoughts occupy most of my time?

What activities occupy most of my time?

How much time is spent bingeing?

What types of activities do I now do to help me cope with stress, conflicts, difficult emotions?

How much time is allotted for growth and development?

How much time do I spend alone, with others?

Is this time enjoyable? Fulfilling?

How much time is spent on activities that challenge and excite?

What are these activities?

How many of my day's activities would I rather not be doing?

When you've finished answering the above questions, again be still and quiet and let yourself feel into the quality of your life at present.

Now, pick a time in your future when you no longer have a problem with food. Again, experience a typical day. Let it be an ideal day. You can have anything you desire in your life. What is it? Where are you living? Who with? What work are you doing? What leisure activities? What foods do you eat? Feel into the overall quality of this life. Take time to write answers again to the questions you've already answered in the first part of this exercise. Be sure to let yourself be quiet and feel into the quality of who you have become. In stillness and quiet, move in consciousness back into the present. Feel the shift in sensation. Again, move into your future. Keep moving back and forth until you feel certain you have registered the differences. What are those differences? How have you changed? Be sure you understand at a deep level not only how your outer activity has changed, but also how you as a person have changed. Are you more glowing? Expanded? Do you have more energy? Are you more accepting, at peace with yourself?

Now ask for guidance. I like to ask my Inner Self, "What do I need to do at this point in time to help myself make this future life a reality?" Be still and wait. Your answer may come in any form — a feeling, a flash of knowing, a visual symbol, a sensation; or it may come from the outside, at a later date — a statement a friend or therapist might make, an event that alters your way of perceiving. Remain open. The answer will come.

Possibly the most profound problem-solving technique I know when searching for an answer, for a solution, is simply to *ask*.

This has been emphasized in motivational and assertiveness training in the sense that you will never get the sale, the job, the raise, the date, the commitment, etc., if you don't ask for it.

It definitely works in external communications, and it likewise works in internal communication. If you have need of an answer, ask the question. Direct it within, to the multitudes that constitute your personality, to your deep Self. Then let it go, for the answer will inevitably come, in its own time. Just as there are no unmatched positive or negative charges, the impeccable accounting of the Universe does not seem to allow for any unanswered questions.

Sometimes it takes awhile, but usually within two or three days it will filter back into your awareness. While taking a walk, or a bath, or before going to sleep, or while waking up — these are all prime times for guidance to come. The more you ask, the more you'll receive.

If you always have the radio or TV on during these times or are chatting, however, the meaningful information may be lost in the noise. Silence can be a luxury in this culture, but if you value the most valuable line of communication in your life, you will learn to cultivate some quietness.

PART TWO

THE STEPS THAT SET ME FREE

When my illness strikes I am irrational, out of control, capable of spending every last penny, incapable of going to work, devious and uncaring of others.

–July 15, 1976

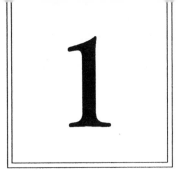

1

Recognizing My Eating
Was Out of Control

Denial

It is so easy to deny this problem. The real issues at hand — dealing with poor relationships, or work and school problems — seem a lot more difficult to handle.

If I focus on my weight, or food, I can keep my brain occupied — and easily measure my success or failure. How to handle loneliness is so difficult a problem, who would want to give up the ease of measuring pounds for the discomfort of feeling empty inside, especially when no tools for handling that loneliness are available? How can we deal with the incredible upsurge of uncontrollable rage that is likely to occur when we first begin to be in touch with anger, especially if there is no way at our disposal to handle that rage? So much easier to stay occupied with dieting. So much easier to measure our progress by the scale each morning. So much easier not to feel the loneliness, the rage. So much easier to eat those ugly emotions away.

No, I don't have a problem with food. All I need to do is lose five pounds, and all will be right. Just a few more pounds, just a few more weeks of dieting — then on with my life.

But, do you ever get on with your life?

No —

Then you have a problem with food!

I had been bingeing for sixteen years before it dawned on me there was something seriously wrong. Up to that point I knew my behavior made me unhappy, but I didn't think I could do anything about it. "Perhaps one day it will go away on its own," I thought.

What made me change?

It was getting worse. I was eating not only at home, in the privacy and secrecy of my four walls, but also on the streets, where I often wouldn't make it to where I was originally headed; at work, where I would search the trash baskets for leftover lunches; at friends' homes, where I would eat their food in the middle of the night; and at night, when I would creep downstairs, slip outside and rummage through garbage pails in the street below my NYC apartment.

In the past, during high school especially, when I would binge I would often cry for help and be consoled by a parent who at least tried to understand me. I would fall asleep comforted by some hope that "mommy" or "daddy" would make it better. Now, living alone, I was left free to eat myself to death, and no one would know. If I was going to get better, I realized I would have to be the one to do it. Weekends spent buried in doughnuts, cake, pretzels, cheese, bread, hamburger meat, ice cream, and bent over toilet bowls disgusted me. I couldn't deny I had a problem any longer.

But what exactly was the nature of that problem? For me, it was simple. FOOD MADE MY LIFE MISERABLE! I had become powerless over the amount of food I consumed at any time of day or night. I had become powerless over the thoughts of food that obstinately and continually plagued my mind. I had become powerless over the feelings of guilt and disgust that threatened to consume every waking moment of my life. I was, in a nutshell, out of control.

I have come to realize that regardless of how often I ate, or how much I ate in one sitting, it was those feelings towards myself that were the issue. The rotten feelings caused by my bingeing seeped into every area of life. I felt hopeless, helpless, worthless, despairing. I discovered that even when I was not bingeing — when I was trying with all my might to control my eating — my life was still being ruled by food. The time I spent not bingeing was just as out of control — and just as miserable.

Feel very sad — binged last night. Not bad, but something wrong inside. Don't want to go through day.

— August 18, 1976

Chances are, if you are reading this book, you think you have enough of a problem with food to warrant trying to do something about it. If that's the case, congratulations! You've taken the first big step. You've realized you have a problem — and are no longer denying it. This is probably one of the biggest steps you'll ever have to take. So, pat yourself on the back and brace yourself for the difficult, but exciting, journey that lies ahead.

EXERCISE

Answer this question: How is food a problem for me? Keep a daily journal and try to stay in touch with how food interferes with your life. At the end of each day, *without judgment*, simply describe when and how you ate, the events preceding any binge, what you might have done if you hadn't binged, and your feelings before, during and after your binge. Also, try to keep track of how often your thoughts go to food — keep a small notebook on hand, and whenever you catch yourself thinking about food (counting calories, craving, planning your meals, berating yourself, etc.), *non-judgmentally* make an entry.

This exercise will help you get objective with your food problem — a way of thinking that will come in handy later, especially when you start dealing with intense feelings. (I talk more about remaining objective in Chapter 7). It will also help you make a deeper commitment to change. Through the process of reviewing your behavior, you will come to know your habits and patterns intimately. This knowledge will help prevent tendencies to deny the problem later, especially when new thresholds need to be crossed.

IN SUMMARY

Realizing you have a problem with food is probably the biggest step you will take, and essential to recovery.

Denial of the problem is easy because it is much easier to obsess about food than to tackle the real but complex issues of relationships, self-esteem, and emotional and creative fulfillment.

If you are reading this book, looking for a solution, for some answers, pat yourself on the back. You have already crossed one of the most difficult thresholds you will have to cross — admitting you have a problem with food!

Wouldn't it be great if all we had to do, as a human race, to be happy and at peace, to avoid World War III, was lose weight? Wouldn't it be great if all we had to do was lose ten pounds each to be promised no more terrorism, no more nuclear fall-out, no more prejudice, poverty, child abuse or illness? Wouldn't that be great?

– June 10, 1985

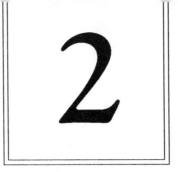

Realizing My Weight
Was Not the Problem

Beauty is One Thing. . . Glamour is Another

Pam is a woman in her early thirties. She has told me she's had a problem with her weight in the past. She's a good worker, dresses well, and looks good. Her weight appears to be normal.

A woman attorney walks into the office. She is thin. Upon leaving, I hear my co-workers discussing her with Pam:

Lucinda: "Boy, I sure would love to be that skinny."

Ginny: "Yeah, she's got a model's figure."

Pam: "Oh, if only I could be skinny like that for just one day!"

Me: "Why?" I scream to myself. "Why would any of these women want to look like that attorney? What is this skinny obsession about?" I want to yell out to them, "What do you really want?"

If only I could raise the consciousness of women, help them go after a life that brings them joy. If you are excited with your life, taking risks, moving forward, changing — you won't care about being skinny! You just won't have time.

But is what I wish for in my life any better? What is the difference? I once wished to be skinny, too. Today I wish to buy land, build a house, start a business, build a family that is close and loving. So, what is the difference between my wishes and theirs?

Maybe it's in the excitement I feel when I envision my dreams. I get a thrill; I'm moved to action. Sure, I have my rough days, but I'm working at what I want for myself, deep in my heart, and this work is nurturing. It gives my life meaning and joy. When all I wanted was to be skinny, it was a wish of despair, not hope. I never believed I could be skinny and so the pain of failure was always with me, keeping me from action — trapped in running circles around an illusion of what I thought would make me happy, but never could and never would. There was no thrill, only the pain of self-hatred.

The trick: let yourself be moved by your desires and set out to achieve them. You will then discover

- there is no need to be skinnier than you are
- you may forget to eat
- it is a waste of time and energy to count calories or go on diets
- it is possible to love the body you have
- others will love you for who you are and the body you have
- you may lose weight anyway but won't really care.

"If only I could lose seven more pounds, then I would be happy!" I cannot even begin to count the number of times I said these words. I was obsessed, as are many women, with the need to lose weight.

Whether I was actually fat is debatable and beside the point. In my mind, I was fat. No one could tell me otherwise. I swore I would make my body thin if it was the last thing I did. Luckily for me, it wasn't.

Looking back I ask, "How could I let such an obsession rule my life?" When I was in the midst of this obsession, however, no one could tell me that what I weighed was not the *real* cause of my unhappiness. I could not have heard those words. I *needed* not to hear those words.

I now know that my obsession was my life-preserver. I was holding on to it for life, and could not let go. If I had, I would have drowned. This obsession had a purpose in my life. It enabled me to stay alive when I had no other way to cope.

YOUR OBSESSION WITH THINNESS IN PART HELPS YOU COPE WITH LIVING. WHEN YOU ARE READY TO FIND HEALTHIER WAYS OF COPING, YOU WILL BE ABLE TO LET IT GO.

Be creative. When the broken record gets stuck at this place:
"If only I could lose . . .If only I could lose . . .If only I could lose . . . ."
— pick up the needle.
Then ask yourself:
What am I really unhappy about right now? Do I feel unfulfilled? Do I feel unloved? Is there something wrong at work or with my relationships? What am I avoiding dealing with? Are there things I am afraid to find out about myself? What about my childhood? Was I an unhappy child? Did this ever really get resolved? What am I protecting myself from? If I wasn't obsessing about my weight, what would I have to deal with?

- going back to school?
- anxieties about graduating from school?
- anxieties over leaving home?
- boredom on my job?
- finding a new job?
- problems with my children?
- problems with my spouse?
- loneliness?
- sex?
- making new friends?
- leaving old friends?
- family crises?
- death?

THIN DOES NOT SOLVE PROBLEMS. THE ONLY "PROBLEM" IT SOLVES IS *FAT*! THAT IS ALL. THIN WILL NOT MAKE YOU RICH, SUCCESSFUL, POPULAR, FAMOUS, HAPPY, IN LOVE, MARRIED, OR YOUNG. THIN WILL MAKE YOU THIN AND THAT IS ALL.

And, there is another side:

WE ARE BEING MANIPULATED EVERY DAY TO BELIEVE "THIN IS IN."

When you watch TV and see a lithe, sexy young girl in a bikini at the beach drinking a diet soda, smiling, surrounded by men, you may think, "Ah, if I were that thin, I, too, could be at the beach surrounded by men, and I too could be smiling. I, too, would be flawlessly happy." Obviously, that is exactly what the soda company wants you to think. If you believe thin is beautiful and happy, won't you buy more Diet Sprite?

See this manipulation for what it is. *Thin* is only *in* because we've been brainwashed to think it is.

FREE YOURSELF!
LIBERATE YOUR MIND!

When you realize you never really had a weight problem after all — you just thought you did — you will be on the road to binge-free living.

* * * * *

I wake up this morning with a sickness deep inside. It has been four years since I've overeaten, and a long time since I've felt this way. I realize that although I no longer overeat, there is a deeper illness that must be cured. It is called despair. Something dark, insidious, comes in on me and causes me to hate my life. I lose interest in everything. Desperately looking for something to make my life worthwhile, I get panicky. The pain gnaws at my solar plexus. I close my eyes and reach deep inside. I travel with my awareness into the pain. It intensifies. I know that if I could get objective to it, I could pull myself out of it, pull myself right side up.

I remember those high school days when this feeling was all I lived with. I woke up in painful despair, living a deathlike existence. I was a compulsive eater then. I blamed my despair on my inability to control my food. Then why, now, do I feel the same despair? I did not overeat yesterday. I did not overeat at all, not at all, during the past year, two years, three years, four! My mind is racing, the pain is gnawing my insides, my mind is working furiously, remembering. Then in a flash, I understand. It is despair that caused the food illness, not the other way around. All those years I was depressed I blamed it on food, but despair was the illness.

Why today, after being healthy for so long, do I suddenly feel overwhelmed and incapacitated? The sickness is still there, eating my insides, paralyzing my motivation. I must take a good look and see it for what it is! It is not me, it is some sickness that comes in and tries to make me think it is me. It tries to make me believe that I cannot do what I want to do. . . that there is no reason for doing anything. . . that all my dreams and visions are nonsense. What craziness this is! I search desperately for the parts that I've come to know as being truly me. These parts find joy and excitement in living. They are filled with visions, and a desire to make those visions a part of my reality. I have enormous power to act and do. I must not let this sickness take this away from me.

I am groping for a larger world. There is an identity crisis. Parts of me are rearranging. With health there comes new mental and perceptual strength and a longing to expand outside myself — to do for humanity what I have done for myself, to help humanity break from the bonds of old limitations and enter new and exciting places. I have come to realize that I am but a microcosm of a world of women existing in a despair that rips off our power. Most women do not know their full power. They accept themselves at 50%, or 20%, or less, of who they really could be. Where does the energy of these women go? Look at the women's magazines! That is where the energy is going. Women are programmed to be concerned with external glamour.

Beauty is one thing, glamour is another. Beauty comes from externalizing inner power. Glamour comes from our need to pretend we are beautiful, a compensation for our own inner fears and weaknesses. Masses of women in the United

33

States are afraid of growing old and dying, afraid of getting fat, afraid of losing the one thing that makes them feel powerful: youth and beauty. With youth and beauty gone, they have lost their power to manipulate.

But true power comes from within. It is a state of consciousness that commands respect regardless of our looks. A woman who knows she is powerful does not need to prove it. As long as we believe glamour is beauty, we will be taken in by a bunch of lies. The glamour magazines make a fortune on this illusion.

As I fight this illusion, I want to help others do the same. You are not alone with your eating disorder. It is a mere mirror of society's value systems. We must fight the mass-mind illusion of glamour by presenting an alternative — real power. We can tap power through continual self-appraisal, constant searching, changing, growing and — above all — a refusal to allow the concepts of glamour to shape our lives.

Glamour thrives on despair. When we are feeling desperate about ourselves, we need to make ourselves feel young, pretty and worthwhile. But when we find real power, we will be creating a world we love, becoming who we want to become, fulfilling the visions we possess, and that beauty will shine through every action we do and every word we say.

I can no longer only act on my own behalf. As I expand, I must grow to include others. That is why I am reaching out to all women. Together, we can change a value system of glamour that pervades our world. If, as a group, we grow away from despair, from fear, into power and understanding of real beauty, we can change the values of our society. As each one of us individually moves through this syndrome, we can create a new order of belief.

— June 8, 1984

IN SUMMARY

"I would be happy if I were thinner" is a false assumption. The only problem that being thin solves is being fat.

However, an obsession with becoming thin will help you cope with living until the time comes when you are ready to find healthier ways of coping.

Your obsession with thinness is not all your doing. We have been brainwashed by the media to believe that "thin is in."

When you realize your weight is not your problem, you will be on your way to binge-free living.

At 6:00 a.m. I wake up and go out and want to eat but refrain and come back and meditate and ask for assistance. I go to sleep and wake up and then go out and stuff myself, craving toast. . .

It is so strange. . . the cravings.

— October 7, 1974

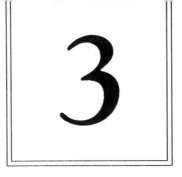

Becoming Motivated to
Live Binge-Free

Making it a Priority

I wanted to be thin so desperately I was willing to do anything to accomplish that goal. I laugh now at some of those things.

In my late twenties I went back home to live with my parents for a couple of years. After dinner my father would wrap a bicycle chain around the refrigerator door and padlock it shut. He would then string another chain through the cabinet handles. I would keep my skimpy breakfast, which consisted of an apple or orange and a hard-boiled egg, outside the refrigerator so I could eat it first thing upon awakening if by chance my father hadn't awakened to unlock the chains. To keep myself from eating this breakfast in the middle of the night, however, I would wrap it in a paper bag and place it outside our apartment in the stairwell. Despite this rather ingenious plan, I was nevertheless able to sneak food out of the refrigerator earlier in the day and hide it close by my bed for my midnight bingeing needs.

So, as you can see, although I tried to control my binges, I discovered that I could not. In fact, the more I tried to become thin by dieting or controlling my food intake, the more I would lose control and despise myself for my weakness. The more I despised myself, the more difficult it would be to stay resolved and committed to my diet. As I became aware that self-control would not work for me, I knew I had to find another way to accomplish my goal.

Instead of resolving again to go on a diet, I decided once and for all to resolve my bingeing problem. I finally understood that I could not prevent those binges with willpower and became determined to find out why they happened and what I could do to stop them. *Binge-free living became my top priority.* Within the time frame of about a year, I did everything necessary to make this goal a reality.

I suppose it is possible to refrain from bingeing indefinitely by overriding the craving for food. But I preferred to tackle the *cause* of the binge — eliminate the craving altogether.

And I discovered that in order to eliminate the craving, I first had to stop depriving myself of the foods I "craved." This meant I had to give up "dieting." In order to stop "dieting," I had to give up my quest for thinness.

But wait! Hear me out. I'm not telling you that you won't be thin. You might very well be thin, and happy too. In fact, I know you will be happier than you are now. At least you will be eventually, because binge-free living is a less stressful way to live. You may have to pass through some less happy times, but in the end, you will be happier — and isn't happiness what we are truly after when we desire to be thin? We think happiness lies in thinness, but we are wrong. It lies in living sanely, in living in control of our lives, in loving, in working, being responsible, being free to be who we are, to feel what we feel, to eat what we want, free of guilt.

It does not lie in secret stashes, lies, humiliation or shame.

If you desire thinness above and beyond anything else, you have what it takes to become binge-free. You have motivation. But, and this is a big b*ut*, you must be willing to allow yourself to let go of that goal, and replace it with the desire to live binge-free.

Please understand that I am not suggesting you cannot become thin once your priorities shift. In fact, I found that as soon as I let go of my desperate desire to be thin and my constant dieting, I stopped bingeing. My body readjusted to its natural weight, and I did lose weight. But, I am not guaranteeing weight loss. I am trying to make a simple point:

NATURAL BODY WEIGHT IS LARGELY DEPENDENT UPON BIOLOGICAL FACTORS. IT IS NOT DEPENDENT UPON YOUR WISHING IT TO BE A CERTAIN WAY.

So, give up. Relax. Enjoy. If you are willing to transform a desire to be thin into a desire to be healthy, fulfilled and at peace with yourself — a desire to live binge-free — chances are you will be happy with the way you look and, if you are overweight, you may lose weight without even trying.

IN SUMMARY

If you want to live binge-free, you must make living binge-free a top priority.

An obsession to be thin leads to dieting, which leads to deprivation. This leads to cravings and, eventually, bingeing.

Natural body weight is largely dependent upon biological factors, not upon your wishing it to be a certain way.

So, replace your motivation to be thin with a motivation to live binge-free. And, if you are overweight, chances are you will lose weight without even trying!

I know I can rid myself of my illness. I know it. But a part of me wants to destroy that knowledge. I know that negativity can be changed into positive energy, I know! But that negativity is so sly and comes in so many varied forms.

— October 10, 1974

Believing I Could Live Binge-Free

Programming to Win. Tools for Change.

When I was a little girl I believed in so much. I could do anything. The world was mine. Then I turned eleven. On the threshold of puberty, things changed. A new self emerged, dark and full of fear. At times when I'd begin to eat, an invisible force would take control. Possessed, I would act in ways I could not understand when I was rational. It was as if I were two people. As I grew, this part loomed larger.

It took me into dark corners, led me into strange alleyways, places I couldn't fathom being when I snapped to. I would do anything to get my fix. Many a night I roamed the dark streets of New York looking for something gooey to shove down my throat. How many wastebaskets did I rummage through? How many hard, stale pretzels did I grab from the garbage bin below my window? How many times did I steal my roommate's food in the middle of the night and have to run out to replace it the next day? How many times did I sneak home late at night, thankful my parents were asleep, so I could lock myself in the bathroom and gorge myself sick? How many times did I vomit in ladies' rooms after lovely meals, feeling guilty because I had eaten a piece of dessert? Was this person the same gifted child who grew up believing she could become somebody in this world?

Yes, she was!

There was something within me that operated below my awareness, that caused me to act in these strange, destructive ways. And yet, there was the other part — the part that grew up believing in a wondrous world of imagination and dreams. I was determined to keep my dreams alive. I was determined to make them a living reality.

COMPULSIVE EATING IS CURABLE! I AM LIVING PROOF OF THAT FACT.

Some people claim overeating is an incurable illness. They are wrong. I fully believe it was the power of my unfaltering desire to hold onto my dreams that gave me the strength to do what it took to succeed.

Last night I ate 2 apples in the middle of the night, so this morning and tomorrow morning I won't have fruit. Today, I nibbled 1/2 oz. farmer cheese for dinner, and half the portion of chicken but some extra farmer cheese. Then getting my period and craving some food, I gave in to eating cole-slaw. Guilt over those few compulsive nibbles, and anger that I am still helpless. I don't like this ridiculous dramatization of my helplessness. I refuse to admit that this disease is incurable and I intend to prove it isn't.

– July 29, 1976

If you believe that you need never binge again, and you are willing to work for it, a time can come when this will be a reality. But it is not just your brain that must believe, it is your whole being — your heart, your spirit. That is not to say you won't doubt. I doubted often. But in the face of my inner knowing, those doubts faded. It was that belief that kept me going, trying, despite constant setbacks.

When my baby learned to walk, he'd fall, pick himself up, and continue on his way as if nothing out of the ordinary had happened. A baby never doubts that he will someday walk — walking is programmed into every cell of his body.

That is the way it is with learning not to binge. After you binge, you pick yourself up and continue on your way. You know you will succeed, and so you continue to do what you need to do to succeed.

Theory has it that as children we are programmed to be and act in specific ways, that our personality and our self-image are molded according to the messages delivered to us by our parents and other important role models. As we grow, we incorporate these messages into our subconscious and proceed to live our lives as conditioned.

If your self-image is low, you will expect to fail. On the other hand, if your self-image is high, you will feel good about what you do and expect to succeed.

If you have a low self-image (as most overeaters do) you can rejoice in the fact that it is not necessary to stay locked in your childhood conditioning forever. It is possible to change. These are some ways:

Four powerful tools you can use to change are positive affirmation, visualization, dialoguing and life-energy. These four tools, when used in combination with one another, will help you make contact with the Inner Teacher and Healer that are aspects of your true Self. The affirmations and visualizations can be used as vehicles through which to activate blocks that must be confronted and transformed if true healing is to take place. The dialogue tool can be a powerful method of finding inner direction, giving new meaning and providing deep insight. Life-energy powerfully alters the conditioned overlays, leaving deep inner essence and transformation. If you are in therapy, these tools can be used to enhance the work you are doing there. If your therapist is unfamiliar with these techniques, you might suggest he/she read this section or any of the books listed below. If you are not in therapy, you may use these tools by themselves, to help you change. However, as these tools can activate painful resistances, it would be beneficial to have a counselor help you through difficult times. Again, I cannot emphasize enough how important it is to realize we each must find our own way to recover. If you have a serious mood disorder underlying your eating disorder, or, if you are taking medication, or you simply do not resonate to this way of working, these techniques may not work for you and that is okay.

(For more information about these techniques, try *Visualization: Directing the Movies of Your Mind* by Adelaide Bry, *Creative Visualization* by Shakti Gawain, *At a Journal Workhop* by Ira Progoff, and *Inner Work* by Robert A. Johnson. Unfortunately, I don't know of any suitable book on the use of life-energy for healing. I am in the process of writing one, however. If you want more information about this, contact me c/o the publisher.)

Let me make it clear that I am not an advocate of the "positive thinking" approach to change. While there is a certain amount of power created initially by affirming or visualizing, I have found that without dealing with the obstacles that are responsible for illness, no real and lasting change will occur. So, while it is perfectly okay to use the dialogue and life-energy tool by themselves, I would suggest you not use positive affirmation and visualization by themselves. In my experience they work much better in combination with one of the other tools.

Affirmations

Positive affirmations are simple sentences repeated over and over again. Some examples are:

"I enjoy learning new things about myself everyday."

"I am a happy, binge-free person."

"As I fulfill my real needs, my need to binge decreases."

To make up your own, first list your needs and wants. For example:

I need:

to be more organized

to see the good in others

to stop bingeing

to become more assertive

I want:

to have more free time

to enjoy life more

Now state each need and want as if you already possess it. Be as specific as possible.

"I am comfortably organized at work and at home."

"I am comfortably assertive about my needs."

"I always see the good in each person I meet."

"I live binge-free easily and comfortably."

"I say 'no' when I mean 'no,' and I state my needs to others in a matter-of-fact tone of voice."

"The leisure time I enjoy balances well with the work I do."

"I get great pleasure from my work and leisure activities, and enjoy the challenges that life presents."

Once you have established your affirmation(s), repeat them at least ten times, twice a day — once in the morning upon awakening and once in the evening, before going to sleep. The more you repeat them, the more power they will have.

Visualizations

Visualizations are pictures you hold in your mind of events you want to occur. Many champion athletes have seen themselves winning in their mind's eye even before the actual event. You can use this tool to visualize yourself doing things in place of bingeing.

For example, imagine yourself being criticized by your boss at work. If a run to the candy machine is something you would normally do, visualize yourself going to your desk, calmly picking up the phone and calling a friend instead. Imagine the phone conversation. What advice are you being given by your friend? Imagine feeling good about yourself for making that call, for finding an alternate way of coping with your insecurities.

Affirmations and visualizations will not work unless they go deep enough to penetrate below the surface of the conscious mind. For that reason the best times to do affirmations and visualizations are when you are totally relaxed and in a meditative state of mind.

I have found that positive imaging always activates its opposite, negative imaging. Do not ignore these negative thoughts and feelings. If you do, they will operate below awareness, and cause you to do and say things you never intended. Here is an example of how this operates: When you say, "Starting today I am going on a diet," this is the positive you affirming future positive action. However, before you know it, you find yourself consuming not just one piece of cake, but two! What has happened? There is a natural law at work here. As human beings we operate in a fashion not unlike a pendulum. When a part of us gets polarized in one direction, another part will polarize in its opposite direction, in order to establish equilibrium. For this reason, as I have said, whenever I practice affirmations and/or visualizations I always work with the "negative" feelings and attitudes that are activated in my awareness. The best tools I know of with which to work these through are "dialoguing" and "life-energy."

Dialoguing

I first learned about "dialoguing" when I attended an Intensive Journal Workshop given by Dr. Ira Progoff in 1974. Although there is much more to his journal process than dialoguing, I had such a profound experience utilizing this tool that it by itself became an ongoing method of resolving inner conflict for me. There are many different ways and reasons to dialogue. For the purposes of this section I will be describing how you can use this tool to understand what motivates your bingeing. (For additional ways to use this fabulous tool, refer to the exercises on pages 47-48.)

Dialoguing helps me understand myself better. When you dialogue with a part of yourself, you are conversing, just as if you were with another human being. You ask that part to express itself, tell you what it is feeling and why. You listen *non-judgmentally*. When it is through saying what it wishes to say, you then respond from your other perspective. I like to think of myself as a house in which live many different individuals with many different needs. When I am in conflict with myself, I find it helpful to have house meetings. Harmony is reached through mutual understanding of the needs of all the members. In this instance there will be essentially two parts of you that will need to meet — the "positive" part of you that you have "affirmed" or "visualized" and the "negative" part of you that has been brought into your awareness. This negative part of you may, in actuality, be many different parts, so be careful to listen to your feelings. They will tell you exactly who wishes to speak and who wants to be at this meeting. You will need to listen to all the parts, letting each speak in turn.

After you have listened to the feelings and wishes of the "negative" aspects of yourself, the "positive" part of you will want to speak. The goal of this conversation will be to come to some form of resolution, through unconditional acceptance of each part's needs. No part should leave this dialogue session feeling unfulfilled. Let's look at an example of how this works.

In this example I repeated the affirmation, "I live binge-free," over and over again. I began to feel uncomfortable and a voice within me spoke:

V(oice) - I don't deserve to live binge-free.

M(e) - Why?

V - Because I'm stupid, mediocre, not worth much to the world.

M - Who told you that?

V - I've always known I can't live up to that grand ideal.

M - What ideal?

V - Being unique, special. What you always tell me I am.

M - But you are unique. You have a lot to offer.

V - What?

M - You have a lot of wisdom. You help people when you offer solutions.

V - Anybody can do that.

M - No. You're wrong. Some people can, yes. But you are one of them.

V - Yeah, but I hate the way you always blow me up to make me seem so great. Then I can't possibly feel as if I can match it.

M - Okay. I understand you feel I make you out to be too much.

V - Yes. Just let me be mediocre for awhile. Let's live with mediocrity. If I didn't feel as if I had to be so great to deserve to be binge-free, maybe I could tolerate it.

M - Okay, even mediocre people deserve to be binge-free.

V - Okay, okay, okay. Now I feel ready to accept it!

When you are dialoguing it is important to let the feelings flow spontaneously from your subconscious. Do not try to control or censor what comes to your conscious mind from deep within.

EXERCISES

Here are some additional ways to use your dialoguing tool:

1. Dialogue with persons: Choose a person from your past or present, dead or alive, with whom you have had or are having some problems. Perhaps you are having trouble with your boss, a spouse, parent, child or friend. After becoming quiet and relaxed, begin your dialogue. You might start out with, "Why are you treating me this way?" or "What do you want out of our relationship?"

2. Dialogue with your conflicting parts: Set up a dialogue between parts of you that are conflicted over something. I like to ask the parts of me that want option (A) to stand over to my right, the parts that want option (B) to stand to my left. I ask my Inner Teacher to stand directly in front of me in the middle. Then I start my debate. I ask (A) to tell its side, then (B) to tell its side. After both (A) and (B) have expressed their views, my Inner Teacher takes over. It turns to each side, asks additional questions and gives insights. Sometimes it sends energy to help heal ideas based on falsehoods or distorted perceptions. There is no way to tell you how to do this exactly or what will happen. In this exercise, the brain is a passive observer. Do not let it interfere with "shoulds" or other preconceived notions.

3. Dialogue with dream imagery: Record a dream upon waking. Choose a predominant image in that dream. Ask, "Who are you to me?" or "What are you trying to tell me?"

4. Dialogue with food: You might start with "Why do I think about you all the time?" or "Why can't I stop eating you once I've started?"

After my dialogue is complete, I like to sit still for a few minutes and think of energy flowing through me and around me, bathing my new selves in healing life-energy.

Life-Energy

The concept of "life-energy" has been around for thousands of years and has been utilized by many cultures. It is used in various forms of martial arts (T'ai Chi, Karate, Kung Fu, etc.) and healing techniques (acupuncture, polarity therapy, Reichian therapy, etc.) and is the inspiration for the "Force" popularized by the *Star Wars* movies.

I first became acquainted with it in Hatha Yoga class where I was taught to breathe "prana" in and out with every breath I took. I later discovered a healing technique taught by a school of Agni Yoga that utilized this energy in its meditation work. In Agni Yoga, life-energy is perceived as "light" energy. When I think of myself bathing in life-energy, I usually experience myself surrounded in a bath of crystal clear light. However, the way you choose to think of life-energy is up to you. Perhaps you experience it simply as a force that gives vitality to living things. No matter. What is important is that you allow yourself to recognize there is a life-force, and that this force has healing properties.

This is really not such an esoteric idea. Healers and physicians from virtually all cultures have known that they themselves do not do the healing. Our own bodies know exactly how to heal themselves with little or no intervention, given the chance. It is the life-force that animates the cells and molecules. It is the life-energy that brings them back into balance, back into wellness.

You can learn to utilize this resource of energy to help heal the parts of you that are mentally and emotionally, as well as physically, ailing. Begin by allowing yourself to take a long bath in this luxurious energy whenever you feel anxious, irritable, depressed, lonely, or hurt in any way. Simply become as relaxed as you can (sitting or lying). Think of this energy surrounding you, flowing in and out with every breath, bathing your inner organs, your thoughts, your emotions. You will feel an incredible release of tension as you continue to work in this way. Working with energy can become a habit. Strive for this. It can change your life.

EXERCISE

(This basic life-energy exercise, along with the dialogue technique, are building blocks upon which further in-depth work is based. I will be referring back to them repeatedly throughout the remaining chapters of this book.)

The technique described below (adapted from the teachings of the School of Actualism, headquartered in Escondido, CA) should not be confused with imaginative mind-play or visualization. The "light" described herein should be viewed, rather, as real — it is a term used to describe the very real life-energy present within all of us. With this exercise you will be learning how to tap into, channel and direct this life-energy for healing.

When you think of an energy, it will flow to where you think of it going and will concentrate in those areas. The trick is to then let go of the thought and simply experience what happens within you.

1. Sit comfortably in a chair, feet flat on the floor, hands on your thighs, palms facing downward. Close your eyes and let your mind soften, relax.

2. Think of a point of light floating six inches above the top of your head. (After you think each thought in this exercise, let the thought go, relax your mind and experience what is happening.)

3. Think of the point of light expanding in size to approximately three inches in diameter, becoming a luminous, crystalline white ball of energy. Think of this ball of light opening and showering a great flood of energy. Experience this energy as it downpours through your body and out the bottoms of your feet, cleansing and washing away all toxic debris, leaving you feeling fresh and clean. Think of your feet closing and experience this great downpour of crystal white light-energy as it starts to backup from below and fill every cell and pore of your body. Let your body soak up this wonderful, pure white light-energy.

4. Sit still with this for awhile and let yourself feel the essence, your purified energy, pouring into every part of you — body, mind, emotions. Slowly open your eyes and observe the changes that are happening within.

EXERCISE

The following exercise is one I do whenever I wish to bring about profound and lasting change. It will help you express what you want to become, through affirmation or visualization. It will help you become aware of the forces within you that are now operating to prevent you from being in that new place. It will give you insight into the reasons for those obstacles and a deep understanding of their purpose and meaning. This, in fact, will help you let go — as you learn to understand and forgive. And, finally, it will provide a real method of transforming those obstacles, through the channeling of life-energy.

1. Get into a comfortable position, with pen and paper on your lap. Close your eyes. Breathe deeply. Relax.

2. Start your affirmation or visualization. Repeat your simple affirmation as many times as necessary. If you are doing a visualization, imagine every detail of the event, how you feel, the qualities you possess. To help you get started with your visualizations, make a list of some of your most vulnerable times of day. Now, make a corresponding list of things you could do at those times instead of binge. Pick one item from the list, close your eyes and imagine yourself in the tough situation. Feel your anxiety increase and the desire to binge come over you. In your imagination see yourself remove yourself from the triggering situation and take an alternative positive action. Live every detail of that event. The more sensory and emotionally vivid it is, the more powerful the visualization event will be.

3. Become aware of the doubts and fears that surface. Do not repress them. They are part of you and need to be integrated and accepted.

4. Explore those doubts and fears fully. What are they telling you? Are they saying, "I'm not worthwhile enough to live without bingeing," or "I would be too sexually attractive," or "What would I do with my time?" or "I would have to deal with loneliness." Keep exploring and write down all your thoughts and feelings.

5. Accept these feelings — they are a part of you.

6. Dialogue with these feelings.

7. Bathe yourself in healing life-energy.

IN SUMMARY

Believe in your dreams. Never stop trying to make them a reality.

Believe that compulsive overeating is a curable illness. I am living proof of that fact.

If you truly believe you will never binge again, and you are willing to work for it, a time will come when this belief will become a reality.

Four powerful tools to use for change are affirmations, visualizations, dialoguing and life-energy.

If you are in therapy, use these techniques to enhance the work you are doing there. These tools can activate painful resistance and, for that reason, do not be afraid to ask for help. But remember: each of us is on our own personal path of recovery. These techniques may not be right for you. That is okay. The important thing to learn is to trust your own inner sense of direction and wisdom.

Always perform the four above tools in a relaxed and meditative state of mind.

Positive imagery always activates its negative corresponding imagery. Do not ignore or repress this. Use your dialoguing tool to deal with it instead.

Surround yourself in life-energy for healing.

Dream: Vomiting, eating yogurt and blueberries. Trying desperately to find toilet to vomit in. People walking in on me. I give up and say, "Yeah, I'm vomiting, don't care any more." But the food won't come up and I have to confront the fact that I've eaten. The desperation of not wanting to face that fact, the horror.

— August 22, 1976

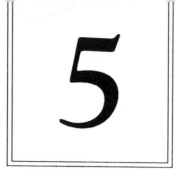

Developing a Healthy
Attitude Toward Food . . .
One Step at a Time

Go Forward Gently with Love. Would a Food-Plan Benefit You?
Setting Up a Reward Program. Four Steps. Reasons Not to Diet.

Each minute I wanted to binge I said, "Jane, just get through this next minute!" Somehow, I could do it for that one minute. The minutes added up and soon it was time for my next meal. I was in heaven.

Then came the end of the meal, and I desperately wanted to keep chewing and swallowing. "How could I stop eating now?" I thought. I did. But just for that minute. Perhaps I made a phone call or read in my prayer book. Soon the minutes rolled into hours and it was dinnertime, when my love affair with food would begin again.

There was something consoling in the idea of "just one more minute." It made anything possible. In time, the minutes became days, days became weeks, weeks became months, and months became years.

YEARS ARE MADE OF MULTITUDES OF MINUTES.
YOU CAN DO ANYTHING FOR JUST ONE MORE
MINUTE.

The only reason we must deal with our food at all is that it has prevented us from making contact with our true Self by handicapping our ability to know and recognize the real issues at hand. If you are not ready to make behavioral changes in the way you eat, no amount of trying will succeed. Remember, bingeing is a badly needed coping mechanism, and you must be psychologically ready to let go of this behavior. If you are not, that is okay. The key to making any permanent change is patience, persistence and self-love. Do not force yourself to do what you are not ready to do. Go forward gently with love.

I now know my bingeing was due to an inability to cope adequately with life's stresses. I had trouble dealing with my feelings, and for that I had to learn new ways to understand and handle my emotions. I had to learn new coping skills. I had to make a commitment to change my attitudes and perceptions. I had to find alternate ways to nourish and fulfill myself — in my work, my creativity and my relationships. But even that was not enough. Although I had been growing and changing in the above mentioned ways for over two years, it was not until I made the decision to *change my food behavior* that I began to see changes in that area as well.

This section describes the physical steps I took over a three-year period that enabled me to finally let go of bingeing and become, in the end, a healthy eater. They were:

- I committed myself to a daily food-plan and eliminated foods that triggered binges.

- I eliminated the food-plan, resumed eating my trigger foods one at a time and made a commitment not to vomit if I binged.

- I did not diet. I listened to my body and ate what I wanted, whenever I wanted.

- I now naturally limit refined flours, sugars, and processed foods, but I never deprive myself of anything.

THERE IS NO RIGHT OR WRONG. SOME THINGS WORK AND SOME THINGS DON'T. THE WAY TO FIND OUT IS BY TRYING.

While you read this chapter ask yourself, "Will this work for me?" Learning to listen to yourself and to act on your feelings is part of the growth process. If you are wrong, you will know through experience. I stumbled along and failed a lot, but I know that through my failure, I grew. I learned by my mistakes. And when I succeeded I had only myself to congratulate. My self-esteem soared. When you fail, ask yourself why. Then give yourself a pat on the back for taking the risk and learning from it.

My First Step:

I committed myself to a daily food-plan, and eliminated foods that triggered binges.

If you can avoid going on any sort of food-plan, do. I am not an advocate of dieting or any other form of controlled eating (as you will come to see by the end of this chapter) unless its purpose is to help you confront emotional issues by freeing up time otherwise spent eating or thinking about food.

When I joined OA I found peace of mind because it gave me a *temporary* way to handle my out-of-control eating. For the first time in my life, I was free to live for days, sometimes weeks, and later, even months, binge-free. I was given a very strict food-plan to follow. It called for a measured amount of protein and vegetable at each meal with nothing in-between and eliminated all carbohydrate rich foods. I wrote down my next day's food-plan each evening before I went to bed and called it into my sponsor. Each evening when reporting my next day's plan, I also reported on how well I had stuck to my plan that day. Writing the plan helped avoid confusion as to what I was supposed to eat and when. When breakfast came there was no room for "Well, maybe just this once I'll have a danish," or at noon, "I'll skip lunch altogether and save the calories." There wasn't any way I could hedge around the fact that my menu had already been structured for me, by me, the evening before.

(A Note: If you do decide to follow a food-plan, however, do not eliminate carbohydrates, as I did. Looking back on my recovery, I now realize that while I did achieve many weeks, and sometimes months, of binge-free living while I was on my rigid food-plan, it was not until I re*incorporated carbohydrates back into my life*, that I succeeded in remaining binge-free. In recent years, research has shown that carbohydrate deprivation can lead to bingeing, and that the consumption of complex carbohydrates – whole wheat, brown rice, buckwheat, oats, corn, barley, millet, potatoes, beans and peas, etc. – is important for optimal health.)

Abstinence first and then start dealing with emotions. Cannot work with emotional states while intoxicated with food!

— March 4, 1977

I love abstinence. I feel so clean and clear in the morning. I love the way my body feels after a week. No worries and cluttered brain with food. I am in touch with what's really going on with me — clarity. Free of food worries, there is serenity.

— November 17, 1979

Although I do not advocate following food-plans, in general, I believe *there can be a time and a place for a temporary food-plan*. Before I chose to follow the food-plan, my days and evenings were so consumed with bingeing that I had no time to explore why I was acting the way I was. The only way I found to free up time and to gain clarity of mind, was to commit myself to a temporary plan.

When I started eating three pre-planned meals a day, for the first time in my life, I had empty between-meal time. I had time to feel lonely, angry, depressed, bored — and I had time to think. Without it I would not have been able to carry out most of the other actions necessary for my recovery.

In one important way this food-plan was different than any former attempts at dieting. On previous diets, I could obsess about what I was going to eat or not eat. On this plan, the most time I spent thinking about what I was going to eat and not eat was after dinner when I was writing out my plan for the next day and calling it in to my sponsor. The parameters of my plan had already been defined by committing them to paper, and my mind was free to think about other things. My feelings began to surface, and I had to start dealing with who I was as a human being emotionally, mentally and spiritually.

Would a food-plan benefit you?

If you have tried a food-plan and still find yourself obsessing about food, following a food-plan may not be the best method for you. Some people need to start dealing with emotional issues *before* they start a plan. If you have had trouble with food-plans in the past, that is okay. Food-plans simply do not work for everyone. If you have never tried a plan and would like to try one, consider the following advantages and disadvantages.

Advantages

- Frees up time otherwise spent in eating and obsessing. This results in increased time for self-exploration.
- Relieves stress caused by fears of gaining weight.
- Gives one a sense of being in control of one's eating habits, thereby resulting in a temporary increase of self-esteem.

Disadvantages

- Deprivation leads to craving which, in turn, leads to bingeing.
- A low-calorie plan can put the body into a "semi-starvation" state. This can result in low energy, mood swings, irritability, cravings and eventual bingeing.
- Keeps you from learning to listen to your own body signals. Decreases body wisdom.
- Can result in a long-term decrease of self-esteem.

If you do decide to follow a plan, keep these points in mind:

- Your plan should be nutritionally well-balanced and allow for variety.

- Include complex carbohydrates in moderation.

- DO NOT skip meals.
  If you skip a meal you will be psychologically and physiologically setting yourself up for a binge. Numerous studies have proven over and over again that people who skip meals during the day tend to binge more at night. This was definitely true for me.

- DO NOT eat *less* than you committed to.
  The same reasoning holds true here. If you deny yourself food, you will be psychologically and physiologically setting yourself up for a binge.

- DO NOT make up for a binge by eliminating your next meal.
  You *must* continue with your plan as if you never binged. If you react by depriving yourself of your next meal you will be perpetuating the diet/binge cycle. In order to break this cycle, it is important to eat your next meal as if you never binged.

57

- DO NOT put yourself down if you binge.
  Remember, bingeing is one method of coping. It is okay to binge. When you are ready to let go of the behavior, you will. In the meantime, do not deprive yourself of your next meal. That is a form of punishment. Instead, try to understand why you binged. Along with examining your feelings, ask yourself if your food-plan is too rigid. A food-plan that is too restrictive can set you up to binge. Be kind to yourself, cherish and trust your own wisdom.

Because, as a compulsive eater, you are probably out of touch with your body wisdom, in the beginning I recommend you seek help in structuring your food-plan. Consult a physician, nurse, nutritionist or therapist familiar with eating disorders. Allow him/her to help you decide upon a nutritionally sound and moderate plan.

Following a food-plan can be a rewarding experience but only *if* you do it in the right frame of mind.

- DO NOT make weight loss your goal.
- DO learn from your mistakes — especially if you binge.
- DO use your "free-time" for self discovery.

My Second Step:

I eliminated the food-plan, resumed eating my trigger foods one at a time, and made a commitment not to vomit if I binged.

Project: To get to source of food problem, both the eating and the vomiting and TO BE FREE OF IT! To rid myself of all hate towards my own body. To eat from inner knowing of what my body wants and needs. To stop eating according to a plan. To enjoy eating, make it a perceptual sensory delight.

Method: Channel love into areas of body I dislike. Acupuncture. Keep daily record of what I eat, and the mental and emotional state I am in when I eat, before and after. Watch my emotional and mental concepts directed towards my body. Before I eat, ask Inner Teacher what to eat and how much. Experiment with foods for their sensory delight.

– June 27, 1978

<u>morning:</u>
1/2 cantaloupe. Glad I had only what I had in middle of night and not more.
Regret. 1 of Kathy's brownie's. Double guilt. 1) at it being hers, 2) at my eating
it at all — but I thought it would be cleaner than eating only a part of it. That
would look like a rat ate it. Hate myself and brownie and Kathy for having it there.
Thinking of going jogging so I don't get fat. Fear and worry.
1/2 yogurt. Tasted good. Sensory delight. Conscious of letting-go of anxiety over
sugar. Hole in stomach.

<u>lunch:</u>
large salad. Very hungry. Eat as I make it. In hurry. Finish feeling good and full.
Ask to make this good for body — cells and organs, and that this food make my
body beautiful, a living temple for my soul.

— June 29, 1978

As time went on and I became psychologically stronger, I began to feel I was ready to try to let go of my food-plan and take trigger foods back into my diet. I proceeded slowly and with caution, testing a tiny amount of trigger food, one at a time. When I decided I was ready to let go of the food-plan I became terribly frightened of gaining weight. A million questions raced through my mind. How would I know when to eat? What would I eat? How much? Would I overeat? Would I binge? Would I vomit? Would I get fat? I was terrorized. I had never eaten without some sort of plan unless, of course, I was bingeing. I had never eaten spontaneously without eventually succumbing to a binge. What was I going to do?

Then I had an idea. I agreed to pay my fiancé $10 each time I vomited. It worked! (This will not work for you if you are not ready to let go of your addictive behaviors. The best time to use this tool is when you have worked through most of your psychological need for bingeing, when bingeing becomes nothing more than an unwanted habit.)

Setting Up A Reward Program

Decide on a prize for behavior you wish to reinforce. Every time you successfully act the way you prefer to act, reward yourself. This prize can be points, money, a material gift (that dress you've been wanting) or an activity (a trip out of town for the weekend, or an hour with your favorite masseuse). Working with points can be creative and fun, too. Assign points for different activities. An example might be: every day that goes by without a binge is worth ten points; every time you refrain from depriving yourself of a food you want, you get five points. When you reach 1000 points, you owe yourself the grand prize —a membership at your local health spa, or that new couch you've been wanting to get for your living room.

If you set up this program with another person, they will reward you for your preferred behavior, rather than you rewarding yourself. (They could offer you a financial gift, or a gift of deed, such as breakfast in bed, a night out, a week's worth of chores.)

Decide on a punishment for behavior you no longer wish to indulge in. An example might be: give away $5 each time you binge, or minus your point count by twenty points each time you binge, and by ten points each time you deprive yourself of something you really want to eat.

If you use money in your program, it should be an amount that you can afford to lose but not so small that it won't deter you.

If you decide to implement a program like this, keep the following in mind:

- Bingeing has a function in your life. Only use this tool if you are psychologically ready to let go of bingeing behaviors.

- DO NOT REWARD yourself for weight loss. If you want your body to weigh less than your body wants to weigh, this method will fail. (This is called the setpoint theory and I'll discuss it at more length later.)

- DO NOT REWARD yourself for depriving yourself of certain foods. Again, if you deny yourself foods your body needs, you will be setting yourself up for a binge down the road.

- DO REWARD yourself for not bingeing, not vomiting or not taking laxatives, but only if you feel you are ready both physically and emotionally to let go of these behaviors — that is, if you have incorporated other ways of coping into your life.

I remember my last binge. I called my fiancé at work to tell him what I'd done and get his support. I needed to hear that it was okay and I did not have to vomit — that he still loved me. I lay there on the bed, stuffed, with tears in my eyes, afraid of becoming fat. His voice was calm and loving. I lay there listening to him tell me it was okay. I soaked the words in. They must have entered my soul because I got off the phone and cried like I'd never done before.

I forgave myself. I transferred his words of love to myself. I loved myself for what I had done. That was my turning point.

When I dropped my food-plan, I was excited about the future, but I was also apprehensive. I was leaving something that I had come to depend on for safety. I was entering an unknown stage of my life, and I was scared.

There was both anxiety and relief in knowing I could order anything at a restaurant, eat at parties and nibble in-between meals if I wanted. My friends tell me I was difficult to be around, especially around food. I would "freak out" if the restaurant put dressing on my salad (instead of on the side) or put butter on my baked potato, and I would find myself frantically scooping out the unmelted butter to escape the calories while yelling at the waitress who was seemingly responsible for that deed. For a long time, when a recipe called for sauteing I would skip the oil and throw the vegetables directly into the pot. I didn't eat croutons on my salad. I never buttered my vegetables. I didn't really know what I could eat or how much I could eat to maintain my weight. It took some time to find out.

My Third Step:

I did not diet. I listened to my body, eating what I wanted, whenever I wanted.

Although I did not binge again, my eating was far from normal. I ate in fear. I ate with control. It took another two years before I felt completely comfortable with food. It took time for me to relearn how to eat — to listen to my body signals and respond appropriately.

Reasons Not to Diet

Dieting Messes Up Your Natural Appestat

During those years of dieting and bingeing, if someone had said to me, "Jane, just eat when you're hungry and stop when you are full," I would have had a good laugh. I didn't even know what being hungry felt like. I didn't know what being full felt like either. I only knew what being stuffed felt like. Needless to say, I had to learn. All those years of dieting and bingeing had messed up my own appestat so badly, it took a while to get it back in working order.

I believe the body has its own wisdom, that if you learn to listen to it and follow its direction, you can do yourself no harm. If you learn to eat when your body tells you it wants food, if you learn to eat the type of food your body is telling you it wants; if you learn to stop eating when your body tells you it has had enough, you will have proper nutrition, you will function at a good energy level, and you will maintain a proper weight.

As I said, it took me awhile to learn how to do this. When I eliminated the food-plan from my life, I began learning how to eat spontaneously. I would estimate it took me (coming from a severe eating disorder) a full three years before I became completely comfortable with eating this way. It might take you longer, or it might be possible for you to do this in a shorter period of time, but you must be willing to risk gaining weight in the process. If you are afraid of gaining weight, you might not allow yourself to eat what your body is telling you it wants.

I know one thing for sure — when I no longer had a repertoire of forbidden foods, I eliminated one powerful source of craving.

EXERCISES

1. Hunger. Fast for a morning, or for as long as you feel it is necessary to empty your body of food. Write down how you are feeling. Do you suspect any particular sensations to be hunger? What are those sensations? A grumbling in the stomach? Weakness? Dizziness? When you suspect you are a little hungry, let yourself go longer. Now what sensations do you experience? Light-headedness? Irritability? Keep doing this until you are so hungry, you know you *have* to eat. At this point ask your body what it wants. Close your eyes. What image pops into your head? Is it a banana split? A hamburger? A salad? A baked potato? Whatever it is, go for it. How do you feel after you've eaten? Are the suspected hunger sensations still present? Which ones have subsided? Make a note of them.

2. Satiety. When you begin eating your next meal, be sure you are hungry. Jot the hunger sensations down in your notebook. As you begin to eat, eat very slowly. Write down how you are feeling as the meal progresses. When you are halfway through the meal, stop. Are the hunger sensations still present? Which ones are, which ones aren't? Ask yourself if you would feel satisfied to get up and walk away from the meal now. If the answer is yes, then do it. If the answer is no, ask yourself why, and jot that answer down in your notebook. Are the reasons emotional, psychological, or physical? If they are not

physical reasons, then know you have satisfied your physical hunger. Give yourself permission to stop eating and to find ways to satisfy the emotional and psychological parts of yourself that are hungering. If you do not want to do this, give yourself permission to eat past your physical satiety without guilt. Do not beat yourself up for it, just be aware you have other needs that call for your attention as well.

3.   Thirst. Next time you think you feel hungry, drink a glass of water instead. Are you still hungry? Or has the hunger been satisfied? Often, we mistake thirst for hunger. I found that I can be satisfied for a couple of additional hours if I drink a glass of juice.

Dieting Lowers Self-Esteem

Why do you diet?
You say, "To lose weight."
I say, "Think again."
If you are overweight (or think you are), and if you are sitting in a restaurant and order a rich dessert because that is what you want, do you feel self-conscious? Do you feel that people are saying to themselves, "Look at that fat woman eating that rich dessert. No wonder she is fat. She *should* be able to control herself!" Don't you feel more accepted, more worthy, if you are at least trying to lose weight? Then people will think, "Look at that fat woman, at least she is dieting and trying to lose weight."

If you are not overweight, you may diet as a preventative measure. Maybe you were once overweight and are still conditioned to behave and think as if you still are, or your parents were overweight and you diet so as not to suffer the ridicule they did. Maybe you are not overweight, but somehow perceive yourself to be, or fear getting that way. Whatever the reason, all dieters have one thing in common. Dieters feel unworthy – they diet to make themselves feel better. ✳

Very few people diet for health reasons. If health were the motivating factor, why would people go on ridiculously unhealthy crash diets, use amphetamines, have their jaws clamped shut, their stomachs stapled?

If you suffer from obesity, these feelings of unworthiness are so linked to the way society treats you that it is hard to separate where your feelings of unworthiness begin and end, and where society's projections on you begin and end.

But if your weight is within a "normal" range, the problem of personal unworthiness is easier to solve. You must first realize your problem comes from within you. When I finally came to understand this and improve my self-esteem, my need to diet decreased.

The way you feel about yourself is the way you project yourself to others. If you feel ugly, chances are you wear unbecoming clothes, your posture is slumped, and you avert your eyes when you speak. Who could blame others for thinking you are ugly? Then, if people say, "What an ugly, fat, individual that person is," you think to yourself, "See, I knew it; my fat is ugly, and their remarks prove it." But if you accept and feel good about yourself, wear stylish clothes, stand erect and look directly at others when you speak, people might say, "She sure carries herself well, I respect her for her self-assurance. I wish I could feel that good about myself."

You can feel good about yourself no matter what you weigh! Dieting is an inappropriate tool for increasing self-esteem. Here is why.

• **Dieting undermines decision-making capability.** Dieting makes you dependent on what others tell you to eat and not to eat. Faith in one's own ability to make even simple decisions is greatly diminished. How can you believe in your ability to tackle some of the greater problems of life, if you can't even decide what you should eat for breakfast?

• **Dieting creates a failure complex.** 98% of people who diet fail! If you are one of that 98%, you have a good chance of suffering from a failure complex. You've probably dieted more than once. How many failures do you think your fragile ego can take before it begins to feel less than human? If you are one of the lucky 2%, you can ignore this point.

• **Dieting = poor nutrition = poor performance.** If you are a chronic dieter, your health has undoubtedly been impaired. It is difficult to function well physically, mentally or emotionally when nutrition has been hampered. Recent studies have been done which show malnourished people suffer from a preoccupation with food, lack of energy, poor concentration, increased irritability, apathy, depression and anxiety. If you are not functioning up to par because of poor nutrition, no amount of therapy will be able to help your wounded ego!

• **Dieting leaves little time or energy for self-development.** When your energy is involved in calorie counting, and other types of food obsessing, there is little time or energy left for activities that bring you pleasure. You then miss out on those wonderful feelings of prideful accomplishment which those with high self-esteem get the pleasure of experiencing.

• **Dieting encourages self-hatred.** In essence, when you diet you are saying to yourself, "I don't like you the way you are. I only like you when you are thin. Do not expect any love from me until you prove yourself to me!" If a friend of yours said that to you, would you still consider that person a friend? I wouldn't. I expect my friends to accept me the way I am. It's pretty difficult to experience high self-esteem when you can't even be your own best friend.

Here are things I did to help improve my self-esteem:

- **I acknowledged my accomplishments.** Each evening before I went to bed, I made a list of the things I did that day that made me feel good about myself. These accomplishments were not necessarily big. They were as simple as, "I cooked myself a delicious meal," "I cleaned out my closet," or "I told Mary she looked good today."

- **I stopped negative thinking and replaced it with positive thinking.** When I became aware that I was putting myself down in any way, I'd try to replace that thought with a positive one. For example, if I went shopping for a new dress, and tried on a size 12 which I thought should fit but found was too tight, my immediate reaction would be, "Ugh, Jane you ugly fat thing, you've got to lose weight!" I'd try to catch myself thinking like this and replace it with a more positive thought such as, "Jane, this dress is too tight. It hasn't been cut correctly. Let me find a dress you'd feel better in."

- **I stopped mind-reading.** People with low self-esteem often assume other people are judgmental and critical of them. When a person acts in a way that hurts you, or says something in a way that leads you to believe they are being critical of you, ask the person to explain in more detail what they meant by their behavior. You can also express your hurt and anger to that person in a way that doesn't blame them, but lets them know how you are feeling. I once went for days assuming a friend of mind didn't want her child to come and play with my child because I thought she was angry with me. When I finally brought myself around to asking her about this directly, I found out she had been preoccupied with a death in her family. I had been the farthest thing from her mind.

- **I stopped comparative thinking.** We all like to compare ourselves to others. Perhaps this is a human trait. However, the person with low self-esteem has a tendency to do this in a way that puts him/herself down. Why not try to learn from our comparisons instead? I started taking note of how I compared myself to others. When I found myself doing it in a way that put myself down I'd catch myself and try to see myself in a better light, rephrasing my comparison to help myself grow. Here are a couple of examples: 1) "That woman is so thin and pretty. I feel like such a big fat horse next to her." Change to "That woman is thin and pretty. I am big and powerful. Isn't it interesting that there are so many varieties of form and beauty among us?" 2) "Those people have such a lovely house. Mine is a dump." Change to "Those people have such a lovely house. I wonder what they do that I don't do? I will ask for some advice."

- **I stopped perfectionist thinking.** Many of us have a tendency to set our goals too high. We then hate ourselves when we fail to meet those goals. Perfectionist thinking occurs in those with low self-esteem, who feel they should be able to do things better than the average person in order to make up for the worthless feelings they keep inside. The only way to combat this perfectionism is to learn to accept ourselves for who we are and enjoy our projects no matter what our performance level is. I made a list of the areas in which I was trying to excel. I studied this list and asked myself, "What activities did I truly enjoy doing? What activities made me uncomfortable? Can you see how driving yourself to excel in any of these activities takes the pleasure out of doing them? Study your behavior for awhile. Try to stop your "driving" thoughts. When you notice you are no longer enjoying an activity, ask yourself, "Why?" "Are you worrying?" "Are you trying too hard?" Then say, "STOP", try to relax, breathe and center yourself. Find the pleasure place again.

• **I accepted my imperfections.** Through the repeated efforts of others telling me it was okay to make mistakes, I slowly began telling myself it was okay to make mistakes. It was a slow process but I finally learned to accept my own imperfections and the imperfections of others. I stopped harassing myself over the mistakes I made. I stopped criticizing others for theirs. My favorite slogan has become, "We live in an imperfect world."

• **I learned to accept compliments.** What do you do when you are complimented? Do you say, "Who me? It was nothing really, anybody could have done it?" If you do, you are putting yourself down. Why shouldn't someone give you a compliment, and why shouldn't you accept it graciously? I've learned to say "Thank you" with a smile and leave it at that.

• **I worked at enhancing my body image.** I worked consistently at learning to accept my own body. I got massages. I dialogued with my body. I channeled healing energy into every cell and pore. In short, I learned to love myself. (Chapter 8 includes a section on body acceptance. It contains good suggestions on how to improve your body image. Also, an excellent book to read is *Transforming Body Image* by Marcia Hutchinson.)

• **I increased my pleasure activities.** Many of us with low self-esteem are so used to putting ourselves down and feeling miserable that we've forgotten what it feels like to simply enjoy life. I made a list of activities that gave me pleasure and began incorporating them into my life. I was actually able to forget about food when I was engrossed in an activity I loved to do.

Dieting Makes You Fat! — Natural Weight & Setpoint Theory

Have you heard of setpoint theory? If you haven't, you will. I believe it will be a buzz word of the 90's. For those of you who don't know what it is, let's start with a definition.

Setpoint is the weight your body naturally rests at when you eat "normally," *ie.*, when you are not dieting and not overeating. There is research that now shows the body will defend this weight at all costs.

Have you even wondered why 98% of all people who diet fail? If diets were all they are made out to be, wouldn't you think at least 50% of people who went on diets would keep their weight off? Science is seriously questioning the validity of dieting for weight loss. Studies have been done in which normal weight people have been put on "semi-starvation" diets. People who were once normal eaters become obsessed with food, develop insatiable appetites and *gain back even more weight than the amount they weighed at the beginning.* Science is also finding that the metabolisms of "semi-starved" people actually slow down. Is this an attempt by the body to protect it from too much weight loss?

One theory suggests the body does not know the difference between dieting and true scarcity. In times of famine, those who have more fat survive. The thin ones don't make it. Thus, when you diet your body fights to ensure your survival by 1) slowing down your metabolism and 2) increasing your appetite.

In his book, *Diets Don't Work,* Bob Schwartz tells how he helps numbers of people who cannot gain weight, gain weight. He puts them on diets!

"We put them on this diet for three days. Most of them have a terrible time because they've never dieted and are horrified at the thought of losing more weight. If they stick to the diet for three days, they may lose anywhere from two to seven pounds. At this point their confidence in our expertise hits rock bottom, but then we take them off the diet and allow them to eat normally. Within a few days they've gained all the weight back — *plus some.*

"Soon their weight levels off, and immediately we put them back on the same diet for another three days. This time they lose maybe one to five pounds. They're not as scared this time, because they're beginning to understand. We take them off the diet, and again they gain back the weight they lost, plus some.

"Again we put them on the same diet for three more days, and this time they *don't lose any weight at all.* And when we take them off, they gain. We keep doing this — one step backward, two steps forward — until they're the weight they want to be.

"Sound familiar? Sound like your life? You see, **diets do work — in reverse.** They're the **best method for gaining weight ever discovered.**"

Here one has to ask, WHY? Why is it so difficult to lose weight on a diet? Why do we hit those awful plateaus even though we are starving ourselves to death? Why do we gain back more weight when the diet is over? No one knows for sure, but the facts are enough to persuade me to stay away from dieting. I do know my weight now pivots around the 130 lb. mark no matter what I eat.

I hear some of you saying, "130 lbs.! I'd die if I weighed that much!" I hear others of you saying, "130 lbs.! What I wouldn't do to weigh that little!" But nature is not fashion conscious. There are as many different body sizes as there are different people. How you look is dependent upon your genetic make-up and your lifestyle. Some of us are born short, some tall, some with dark hair, some with light. The variations in our appearances are endless. Why do we expect we should all weigh the same? Setpoint weight varies. For some it may be higher than you wish it to be. For others, it may be lower. The number of fat cells your body carries is largely dependent on heredity. So why fight it? It would be futile to try to be shorter than you are, or taller.

I hear those moans! Please don't despair completely. It is possible to change setpoint. Although setpoint is largely dependent on heredity, it may be possible to alter it through exercise.

But I'm not the expert on setpoint and dieting. I'm only rephrasing what I've read. At the back of this book I've listed a number of excellent sources of literature on this theory. Read the facts for yourself and decide.

My Fourth Step:

I now limit refined flours, sugars and processed foods, but I never deprive myself of anything.

As I became more comfortable with eating spontaneously, my taste in food began to change. In the beginning I was cautious. After many months of experimenting and finding that it was safe, I went through a "junk" food phase. I ate anything I wanted without fear and loved it. A time came, however, when my body began to lose its desire for gooey, sugary, salty things. I started craving more whole foods — vegetables, fruits, protein, and whole grains. Today, my diet consists mostly of these foods. I actually cringe at the sight of a white-bread sandwich. Why not eat a sandwich on whole wheat bread, increase the nutrition you get and give your body an optimum chance at health and high performance?

As there are so many good books on nutrition, I'm not going to talk about it here. I'm not the expert. But I do know that since I've been eating nutritiously, taking vitamin and mineral supplements, and exercising regularly, my health has been excellent, my energy level high, and I feel emotionally and mentally very stable. But remember, I believe in the wisdom of my body, and although I stick to nutritious whole foods most of the time, when my body tells me it wants a refined, gooey goody, I do not hesitate to gratify its request.

IN SUMMARY

In order to change your food behavior, you must be psychologically ready to do so. Do not force yourself to do anything you're not ready to do. Go gently with love.

In order to stop bingeing, you must make the decision to change your food behavior.

How you go about changing that behavior is up to you. You are in the driver's seat.

Learn from your mistakes and revise your plan as you go. Stay flexible.

All dieters have one thing in common. They feel unworthy and diet to help themselves feel better.

Dieting is an inappropriate tool for increasing self-esteem. It
- undermines your decision-making ability
- sets up a failure complex
- leads to poor nutrition = poor performance
- leaves little time or energy for self-development
- encourages self-hatred

Better ways to improve self-esteem are to:
- acknowledge accomplishments
- replace negative thinking with positive thinking
- stop mind-reading
- stop comparative thinking
- stop perfectionist thinking
- accept imperfections
- learn to accept compliments
- enhance body image
- increase pleasure activities

Dieting can make you fat.

The body will defend its setpoint at all costs.

Nature is not fashion-conscious. For some the setpoint will be higher than for others — but it is possible to lower setpoint through exercise.

To maintain proper weight and an optimum energy level
- eat when hungry
- eat what your body wants
- stop when you are full

Optimize health, energy level and psychological well-being by eating nutritious whole foods.

Do not deprive yourself of any foods.

When I take a dance class, I am not simply taking a dance class. For me, dancing is a measuring stick. I go in to see where I stand in terms of the values set for myself. I walk pleased or repulsed. But that is a basic perception that has served the past. It has not helped growth.

The mirror, always a way to assess. To be committed to therapy is to be committed to change. However, not the appearance of change, not a changed action — but to change the very perception that guides all action.

— March 5, 1975

Changing My Belief Systems

What is a Belief System? What are Your Belief System?

One summer day, I walked home from class. I was wearing an old shabby, shapeless t-shirt and a pair of dirty jeans that were at least one size too big for me.

Opening the door, I headed straight for the only mirror I kept in the house. I took a long look at myself, turned to the side, grabbed the waist of my pants, tucked in my stomach as far as it would tuck and felt the space that lay between my skin and the jeans. Content that I hadn't gained any weight, I checked out my hair hanging in my face. "I'm sort of shabby looking," I thought. I pulled my shirt up so I could check my ribs and waistline. Looked good, but then again, this was the best part of my body, never gave me much trouble. I turned around 180 degrees, craned my neck so I could look at my buttocks. Too big as usual. A wave of nausea burst forth from deep inside. I flew into a rage, picked up some empty soda bottles and threw some at the wall. I loved the sound of glass breaking. It was so good to get that pent-up rage out. A couple of more bottles and then before I knew it I was out of control in a screaming, crying, bottle-throwing fit.

No more bottles left, shaking, I paced the kitchen floor. What was it Penny had said to me? She had told me I was beautiful. She had told me my body needed to be loved just as I needed to be loved when I was a little baby, just as I would always need to be loved, all of my future life.

Penny had me get into a relaxed, meditative state. She had me move with awareness into the spaces of my body — into the areas I hated the most. I tried, but I couldn't go there. I was completely cut off from sensing into those areas: hips and thighs. It was like it was all black inside there. It as as if there were a thick lead wall that prevented me from penetrating those spaces.

She told me I had to start seeing a beautiful woman, that I had to bring love into the areas I hated. It was too hard, too painful. I felt sick deep in my guts, but I heard what she had said, and I knew she was telling the truth.

A month or so later, I walked straight to that mirror, took a good look at the ugly thing I saw staring back at me and said "I love you." I could not feel the love, but I had decided to go through the motions anyway. "Maybe," I thought, "if I say it often enough, someday I will believe it."

A belief system is made up of the sum total of our attitudes and perceptions. It is deeply rooted and motivates our behavior, often below our awareness. Behind every feeling or action you can usually find an attitude or perception that causes you to feel or act that way. If you are a compulsive eater, you are guaranteed to have a belief system that directly ties into why you eat the way you do and why you feel the way you do. I discovered I held a belief system that went something like this:

- I am fat.
- I am ugly and cannot be pretty until I lose weight.
- I do not deserve to be pretty.

These beliefs resulted in my feeling and acting in the following ways:

- I hated my fat. I hated myself.
- I dieted and starved myself to lose the ugly fat so that I could be pretty.
- I binged so there was no real chance of losing weight or becoming pretty. I didn't deserve to be pretty anyway.

No one had the guts to say to me, "Jane, you want to be fat so that you can believe you are ugly and undeserving of being pretty." If anyone had said those words to me I would have laughed. "No way, I hate fat. I must become thin and pretty," would have been my retort.

One day, a counselor said to me, "Jane, you really are beautiful. From now on, every time you look in the mirror, I want you to say 'I am pretty' to yourself." "I can't say that," I said. "It is false."

"It is false only because you believe it is false. Once you start saying those words you will start to feel differently about yourself."

I went home and started this ridiculous routine of looking in the mirror at this incredibly ugly, fat thing and saying, "Jane, you are really pretty." What a shock that was. I would say those words, then go straight to the refrigerator and binge. No one, not even my own words, was going to disprove my belief system.

As I continued to say those words on a daily basis, I began to realize that there were *parts* of me that needed to be fat and ugly because they felt ugly and lacked love. They could not tolerate the words, "Jane, you are pretty," because they were unable to believe it for themselves. When I acknowledged these parts and used my dialoguing tool to communicate with them and help them, I began to change.

Belief systems are difficult to recognize and change because they are so much a part of us. Change is scary. It can feel unsettling, like losing a best friend, and even though we've outgrown that friendship, we will grieve a loss. Although this feels disorienting at first, in time we will come to feel comfortable once again in our new identity.

To help you begin to recognize and work with your beliefs, I have listed ten beliefs that are common to the compulsive eater.

1. I am fat and ugly.
2. I will *always* be fat and ugly.
3. I cannot control my intake of food.
4. I do not deserve to feel good about myself.
5. I cannot eat over a certain number of calories without gaining weight.
6. If I stopped counting calories, I would be unable to control my weight.
7. I must diet in order not to gain weight.
8. If I have one piece of cake, it's all over.
9. I can't keep "fattening" food in the house.
10. What! Enjoy food? Impossible!

I used to believe every single one of them. I no longer believe any of them. A miracle, you say. No! It just took some work to acknowledge that I had them and to change them. These are the beliefs I operate under today:

1. I am pretty.
2. I will always be pretty.
3. Food doesn't need controlling.
4. I deserve to feel good about myself.
5. I can eat any number of calories without gaining weight.
6. I never count calories; my weight is stable.
7. I never diet and do not gain weight.
8. I can eat a piece of cake (or any of my once "forbidden foods") without bingeing or feeling remorseful in any way.

9. I can keep any amount or kind of fattening food in the house without feeling threatened.
10. I enjoy my food.

YOU MUST CHALLENGE YOUR BELIEFS. THEY WILL NOT COME UP TO YOU AND SAY, "I AM A FALSE BELIEF; YOU NEED TO LET GO OF ME AND FIND ANOTHER." THEY DO NOT OPERATE THAT WAY. THEY STAY GLUED UNLESS <u>YOU</u> MAKE THE EFFORT TO UNGLUE THEM.

REMEMBER THIS: YOU ARE WHAT YOU BELIEVE!

EXERCISE

Make a list of your beliefs. If you have difficulty, start with the list I made and add to it. Go down the list. Say each one out loud. Most often you will know instinctively whether a statement is one you believe in or not. If it is, challenge it.

One good way to challenge the statement is to write down its opposite. For example, if you believe, "I am fat and ugly," then write down on a piece of paper, "I am thin and pretty." The latter statement becomes your affirmation. Say this sentence out loud a few times. Listen to the negative feelings that are activated within you. Keep repeating it. Dialogue with these "negative" feelings. Surround your beliefs and feelings in healing life-energy. Here is an example:

1. The words "I am pretty" become my affirmation.
2. These words activate the parts of me that feel ugly. I acknowledge these feelings.
3. I ask that the parts that feel ugly stand before me and proceed to talk with them. They tell me what they are feeling and why. They tell me they need my continual support and approval.
4. I sit still with these parts a few minutes every day. I send them words of love and surround them in life-energy. As they begin to feel loved, I begin to feel loved. As the parts within me begin to change, the total me begins to change.

IN SUMMARY

A belief system is made up of the sum total of our attitudes and perceptions. It is deeply rooted and motivates our behavior, often below our awareness. Behind every feeling or action you can usually find an attitude or perception that causes you to feel or act that way.

Belief systems are hard to recognize and change because they are so much a part of us.

You must challenge your beliefs. They stay glued unless you make the effort to unglue them.

Make a list of your beliefs.

To challenge the belief, write down its opposite.

Use your dialoguing tool for change.

Remember this: YOU ARE WHAT YOU BELIEVE!

This is the way I see it today – I took Cajun and Annabelle to the doctors. I also spoke with Steve and told him to read some poetry — and I told him that I and Cajun and Annabelle were going to go to the doctor's. I felt no anger. I wrapped them up and the three of us went to the bus stop and there I cried for you. I felt a little angry and then I wrote a poem. I called the poem Murderer after the me that was, and the me that isn't, and the me that felt no anger — only love for you and my friends and Cajun and Annabelle and the green tower.

I boarded the bus and held the box that held Cajun and Annabelle. I held it tightly and read Blake and that is when I wrote the poem called Murderer.

I am on the edge of rage. I am peaceful and inspired. I try to guard against it — I feel it sneak up upon me. I toss it aside and then I pace and a glimpse of newness. I do not have a name! The rage — Steve, how dare you for leaving me!

Rage Rage go away. Don't come back another day.

– May 7, 1973

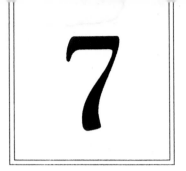

Exploring My Feelings

Rage. The Feelings Diary. Self-Denial. Acceptance. Managing Your Feelings. Loneliness. Expressing Anger. Managing Anger.

Rage! That endearing emotion. How afraid we are of it. Understandably so. It is a powerful one. Rage should not be confused with anger — not the same thing. Anger is manageable. Rage is not. I remember vividly the year I opened up and allowed all that rage to flow from me. My Reichian therapist had me rolling my eyes, pounding the bed, screaming into pillows. Soon I was collecting old glass soda bottles for my rageful glass breaking orgies. If you've never thrown a glass and heard it break, you don't know what you're missing — especially if you can scream at the top of your lungs at the same time. After one of these fits, I usually ended up on the floor, trembling, at peace with myself and the world.

The neighbors? I just told them I was in therapy and had a lot of rage to let out. They never complained. One time, however, the police came to my door. They said they could hear someone screaming and just wanted to be sure everything was okay. "Sure," I said, "everything's fine."

Everything wasn't fine; I was mad as hell. I guess it was all those years of not being nurtured that made me angry, all those years of being denied. Funny thing — rage. It can become a habit. My rage came out of my feeling helpless — helpless for not knowing how to ask for love; helpless at not knowing how to assert my needs; helpless, certainly, at being rejected by Steve. A child is helpless a lot of the time, but as adults, there is a lot we can do to make things better for ourselves — we can learn to assert ourselves, get our needs met, express love and let love be expressed back.

Rage is a child's emotion — deeply felt.

When I started on the food program, eating three meals a day with nothing in between, I suddenly had to cope with the problem of "too much time." I discovered a range of emotions that was both exciting and terrifying. I had succeeded so well in repressing my emotions with food that when I refrained from bingeing, the feelings that surfaced appeared overwhelming.

What I eventually came to know about myself was that I was a depressed, lonely, angry, frightened and self-centered young woman. In a way, it was lucky for me I was a compulsive eater because I had something real against which I could measure my progress. Although my illness symptomatically manifested as an eating disorder, it was in reality a personality disorder. The healing that took place not only required recovery from a food compulsion but also required a full transformation of character.

I had to recover from the despair and the sense of emptiness that filled my life. I had to overcome my fear of others and my loneliness. I had to admit to the arrogance that covered up my low self-esteem. I had to find the rage that was bottled up inside and give it a non-destructive avenue through which to express itself. I then had to learn how to deal with anger constructively. I had to learn to forgive myself and regain my self-respect.

When I first realized I had an illness, I sought only to become a normal eater. I longed for happiness which, to me, meant eating like other people and being thin. Now I know happiness can never come from how one eats. It can only come from how one feels inside.

YOUR FEELINGS ARE REAL. THEY DEFINE YOUR INDIVIDUALITY. IF YOU DENY THEM, YOU DENY YOURSELF.

One good way to become aware of your feelings is to keep a feelings diary. Keep a small notebook with you at all times. Without judgment, log what you are feeling at various times during the day. A few words are all you need. Later, perhaps before you go to bed, you can review your diary and take the time to do your in-depth work. (Throughout this chapter you will find entries I made in my diary between 1973 and 1979. I chose these excerpts to illustrate how I used my journal to focus on a variety of emotional issues. You will see that I experienced much pain, and that although I was hopeful, there were many times I felt discouraged and was unable to stick to my food-plan. I hope these entries will illustrate to you how pain, "failure" and doubt are all part of the healing process.)

This diary is a good way to practice becoming an "observer" of your emotions. Becoming an observer means learning to keep a part of you objective to your feelings. It is the part of you that stays rational, that directs appropriate action.

The more developed your "observer" becomes, the easier it will be for you to realize that "you" are not the same as "your emotions," and it is a lot easier to accept feelings you do not like when you realize those feelings are not "all of you."

I now know without a doubt that my emotions are a part of me, not all of me. I know how to experience my emotions fully without being taken over by them. I know how to keep one foot out of the water, so to speak. The foot that stays on dry land is my observer. It is always objective to what I am feeling. If I am furious at myself for making a mistake, my observer says to me, "Jane, aren't you being a little unrealistic? You are human, aren't you? You are entitled to a few mistakes." If I am angry because my son is overly demanding and I don't seem to have enough time for myself, my observer says, "Jane, your son is in need of something. First, take care of his needs and later make sure you take care of yours." If I awake depressed and do not know why, my observer says "Jane, you need to get breakfast ready, take care of the chores and then make time to dialogue."

My observer takes care of me while helping me to take care of what I need to take care of. Don't underestimate your observer. It is one of your most important allies.

As you continue working with your feelings journal, you will be learning how to accept your feelings non-judgmentally as well.

The painful experience of speaking with my mother is I begin to feel a loss of self — or that I am existent for her, that my wishes and desires are sucked up into her, that what I have chosen to do has all been for her, really — that nothing has been left for me.

— June 7, 1973

Self-denial takes a long time to heal; you have to embrace the slow process of learning who you are. You need time to discard the old, and time to try out the new. I don't ever remember discussing feelings, as a child, just discussing events or outcomes. So, I got my identity from "outcome," not from feelings. This had to change. I had to learn to express my feelings to others and to accept them as my own. I always felt judged because when I did something, it met with either approval or disapproval. It took time to accept the parts of me that were "disapproved" of by well-intentioned parents and time to shed the parts of me that did things I did not want to do because they were "approved" of by well-intentioned parents. I had to learn to become ME in my own right and to shed the identity of the little girl who was the little girl my parents always wanted to have. It eventually took a lot of teenage (and beyond) rebellion to break away and start to find the real me.

Most of us judge our feelings. We think some are good and some are bad. Anger is usually a feeling many of us would rather do without. Because of our low self-esteem, compulsive eaters will go to extremes to be "liked." Anger is not very "likeable," so we prefer to eat rather than express it.

Feeling weak or vulnerable is another distasteful emotion for many. If we expect ourselves to be strong and in control all of the time, we will have a hard time accepting our need for others — the need to be consoled, hugged, to have a hand to hold through a difficult time or a shoulder to cry on.

I had to learn to accept these "difficult to accept" emotions. I learned it was okay to be angry, and it was okay to need others.

What feelings do you have a hard time accepting?

"The Unconscious Binger"

She is standing in front of the refrigerator eating from a container of cottage cheese with her fingers. Her mind is racing. She is thinking about her day at work, about a co-worker. She is feeling increasingly uncomfortable. She reaches for some cheese, her mind still obsessing. She continues to ignore it, eating the cheese instead. By this time she feels disgusted with herself. Her thoughts shift from her co-worker and focus on the food she is eating; she is into a full-fledged binge.

If she were to use her bingeing to track her feelings, the incident could proceed this way:

"The Conscious Binger"

She comes home from work feeling uncomfortable. She heads straight for the refrigerator and opens the container of cottage cheese. She knows something is wrong because she's not yet hungry and had planned to go jogging anyway. This is her cue to watch herself closely. As she eats the cottage cheese, she realizes her mind is racing. The thoughts that are occurring have something to do with an incident at work. Again, this cues her that something is wrong. She says to herself, "Something is bothering me about the incident at work. I need to find out more about it and what I am feeling. I know I'm really not hungry." She then closes the refrigerator door, gets her notebook, sits down and begins to explore her feelings.

Although this works best when you actually experience the desire to binge, circumstance can make this difficult to do. If you cannot stop yourself in the middle of a binge, you can re-enact the scene at a later time and still learn from it. Close your eyes. Re-experience the scene exactly the way it took place. Observe your emotions as the desire to binge overwhelms you. Write down what you were thinking and feeling. Accept those feelings and proceed to work with them.

Now I get memories of sexual attitudes, how can I pretend that I am separate from the vibrations that were felt in my house when I was a child. I carry with me all that in the pockets of my muscles and innards and cells. Somewhere in me, in the depths beneath my consciousness I hate my body. I hate sex. I cannot look at my father. I will betray my mother. Shame on me. And so I made myself ugly and refused to look at him and always hid from him and never opened myself, never could make myself pretty.

I don't want to be free. I can't stand the burden of this responsibility and maybe these insights are too painful. I am in so much pain and I blame him now for not being there to comfort me, to relieve me of the pain.

The child is in a rage because it doesn't want to leave; it is hanging on for life. It is yelling, "Jane, you idiot, you are a good for nothing, how dare you betray your father, how dare you betray your mother and walk the earth without them." Without a mother and without a father a child is left to die. My child is dying and it is screaming and tearing at me.

—May 7, 1974

Dream image:
Talking to my father. I'm standing on top of the staircase banister and am about to fall.

If I can stand up as tall as him I will fall. Jane is still a little child. Stand up tall little girl and talk to him for he will not kill you. Speak up little girl despite your fear, for fear is the illusion that prevents growth. Oh little girl you try to stand on

*top of banisters. You should not want to climb. You need to grow inside instead, to
the height of him — to equal and to speak.*

— June 2, 1974

Once I began accepting my feelings, I needed to find a way to handle them.
It's one thing to say, "Okay, I've accepted my rage," and be fuming uncontrolla-
bly, and another to know what to do with emotional outbreaks. In order to
effectively manage your feelings, it is important to keep two things in mind.

• **Realize that you alone are responsible for your feelings.** I have found
that under no circumstances is anyone ever responsible for how I am feeling. This
was a difficult lesson to learn. So often we want to blame others for our anger,
our grief, our loneliness. Just isn't true! No one makes you angry — you make
yourself angry. When you realize that you are the only one responsible for how
you are feeling, you will also realize that you are the only one who will be able to
change the way you are feeling. Thus, if you feel lonely because your boyfriend
left and you continue to blame your loneliness on "his leaving," you will have a
hard time finding any solution other than "his coming back." This leaves you in
a rather vulnerable and helpless position — it makes you dependent on him to
feel better. But if you take responsibility for your loneliness, you can access any
number of useful solutions. You could, for example, take pride in teaching
yourself to enjoy your alone times. You could spend more time with other friends.
You could take advantage of the opportunity to begin exploring whole new
relationships.

By taking responsibility for your feelings and taking action to change, you
learn to manage your feelings.

• **Magnify your observer.** You have had some opportunity to strengthen
your "observer" muscles by keeping a journal. Casually jotting down a rageful
feeling will not work, however, especially if you feel like throwing bottles. So the
first thing I always do is move into "observer" awareness. That is, I consciously
tell myself that although I am very, very angry, there is a part of me that is not
angry, that is observing this situation and will help me find a more rational
solution to it. I think of magnifying the observer within, and proceed to work
with one of the following tools: (Remember: these tools worked for me. They
might not work for you. Try them a few times. If nothing happens, go on to
something else. Always trust your own instincts.)

• **Tool 1: I discuss my feelings with others.** If my emotions involve
another person, I try to talk about my feelings with him/her. The way another
reacts is often the result of how I've chosen to communicate my feelings. So if
I start yelling and accusing, I am sure to get a lot of yelling and accusing back. But

if I start out by saying, "I'm very angry about what is happening here. Can we discuss it and try to find a solution between us?" I will usually end up in a discussion that is fruitful and mutually beneficial.

Even if my emotions do not directly involve someone else, discussing them often helps me gain clarity and helps me move toward resolution.

- **Tool 2: I dialogue.** Many times we experience feelings that we don't understand. Feelings can appear overwhelming and confusing. This tool has helped me gain invaluable clarity, as well as resolve issues. You might choose to dialogue with the parts of you that feel angry, lonely, sad, confused, whatever. A simple question like, "Why are you feeling so angry?" is all you need to get you going. Continue the dialogue until you feel you have reached a reasonable resolution. Here is an example:

One day, a few months before completing the final draft for this book, I was feeling angry but didn't know why. Mentally I reviewed the events of the past few days but came up with nothing. When I sat down to dialogue, this is what I discovered:

M(e) - What are you so angry about?

A(nger) - So sick of having to prove ourselves. Fed up, in a rage over it!

M - How so? How do you have to prove yourself?

A - Having to be the best. Having to be liked all the time. I'm mad cause I don't want to be the "special" one, put up on a pedestal, it's too painful.

M - Who's making you feel this way?

A - In order for the book to sell, it has to be better, that's screwing us up.

M - You know, you don't have to be *better* to be a worthwhile person, unique and special, and deserve to be read. You don't have to be better to be any good.

A - Then why should anyone read this book? They could just as well read all the others.

M - Yeah, and some they'd like more than others. If I was still bulimic, I'd probably read all I could and take from each what I could. You're special in that you have something unique to offer, but not *better*! Can you handle that?

A - Yeah, we're just so sick of having to fight this low self-esteem all the time!

After this dialogue session I realized that I still had parts of me that were feeling unworthy of publishing a book. They were becoming angry in response to the impending publication date. Through dialoguing I became aware of their existence, and I was able to help them understand it was possible to be unique (and have something special to offer others) without having to be better than every other book. If I had not done this session, my low self-esteem could have eventually sabotaged the completion of this book. My anger could have eventually been directed towards myself. I could have become overwhelmed by depression and unable to complete the book, or perhaps I could have taken on too many responsibilities, causing me to become "too busy" to complete the book. Instead, in becoming aware of the anger and what was causing it, I was able to make appropriate choices. I decided to do what it took to go ahead with the completion of this book despite the parts of me that felt inadequate and to work on healing my low self-esteem.

- **Tool 3: I release.** Sometimes I simply say to myself, "Jane, let's let go of this feeling. I don't want to be bothered." It works.

- **Tool 4: I channel life-energy.** I channel life-energy (see page 49) and think of the feeling being gently washed away, out of my body and into the earth.

- **Tool 5: I channel light-fire.** The following exercise is an example of how this works.

EXERCISE

1. Begin by channeling life-energy as directed up through Step 3 of the basic exercise on page 49.

2. Hold the awareness of the emotion in your mind and think of energy surrounding it.

3. Now think of the energy turning into a great ball of fire, consuming all self-destructive emotions and leaving in their place positive, life-supportive emotional essence. Hold the feelings within the fire until you feel them dissipate. With thought you can magnify the consuming power of the flames.

4. Think of the essence soaking into your entire body/mind. Allow yourself to sit with this positive essence for at least ten minutes before engaging in other activities. Doing so will enable you to more fully assimilate and incorporate the change into your life.

My body completely swollen. Feel fat and bloated, could be pregnant. Crying all the time. Very sexual, no one to love. Seeing Philip yesterday was painful. There is no communication. It's obvious he doesn't want it. I could scream the scream of life and how it alters — Why? Why? Why did it turn out to be like this! My arms ache for love. I can feel the energy in my arms and there is no one here to accept it.

– October 7, 1974

Remember the feelings of Mommy, I want Mommy. Feel bad now about not letting those feelings come out. I didn't go with it. Nausea and fever.

– October 10, 1974

I ate to cover up my fear of people. I was so alone; when I found a man to love, I would cling to him for fear he would leave me. I lived through others — clinging desperately to them for approval. This is not the way to make and keep friends, but I didn't know how to love because I couldn't love myself.

I remember the parties I went to — standing by the refreshment table watching the others talk and dance. Feeling more and more uncomfortable, I'd start to nibble at cheese and crackers, have a drink, take some celery, more cheese; before long I would be eating as much as I felt I could get away with. Stuffing my pockets when no one was looking, I'd make my escape down the elevator, hail a cab, eating all the way. When I arrived home I would continue without inhibition to stuff myself sick! I never once thought to ask myself "Why?" Why did parties make me so uptight? Why was I so uncomfortable around people?

At other times I would hide quietly in my own apartment, until friends knocking at my door went away. I remember turning down social events many times to eat instead. And yet I never knew how lonely I was — not until I started my first food-plan. It was then, without the crutch of food, that I realized how devastatingly lonely I actually was. At times it was unbearably painful; those were the times I broke my commitment with a binge.

I am feeling choked and sad, lonely. I don't like Saturdays. The families and children — I feel left out. Noticed Laura and her friend. How bouncy she is, and happy. I am sad and lonely, send love into these negative feelings. Keep working through tension and pain in heart area.

– October 13, 1974

*Last night I ate like a fiend and had sweaty anxious dreams over the performance —
things going wrong, insecurities. I am very intense and anxious this morning and
fat. Well, at least I know it's fear of not being able to pull this thing off and there is
no real reason not to if I keep a cool head and meditate every day. Oh God — dear
Lord, dear Lord. Whenever I get taken by the appearance of things I'm sunk.
Please help me stay centered — love — it's you I want to know. Only you can lift
me up and out of the realms of pain. Dear God, what must I do to keep you being
close to me even when I am lost?*

— October 21, 1974

*Very important to work out all negativity. I will not be able to proceed without
doing so.*

— January 30, 1975

*Last night it felt strange. I felt strong and in period of transformation. I could feel
the image that was guiding me. I could feel the little girl in me, the little fat ugly girl,
scared to leave home. How much of that image of Jane, the little fat girl, still
breathes inside me? I try to feel what it would mean to live now free from that
image. Who would I be?*

— February 4, 1975

*I see myself at the bar seducing, afraid of the men, my eyes downward. I run from
them. And then I see my whole being looking at each man and saying, "Hello,"
and coming forward and being not afraid, but confronting each and every one of
them as one human being to another.*

An image of looking at a man and seeing his being, not his sexuality.

— July 7, 1975

*Negative forces coming over me. General horrendous emptiness. Eating and
vomiting again all day, and cry, cry, cry, and I realize how blind and deaf I am,
with no internal eyes or ears. They sleep. I do not hear or see with spiritual eyes
and ears. They are not yet opened. I am so sad and in contracted pain and desire
to eat, eat, EAT. But, no! And I will stop letting that pain rule my life. I will
rule it, get behind it. Something wants to be freed and it fights and then the negative
fights to keep it behind bars and my body hurts in my throat and heart. After*

meditating, I am tired and lie down. I see a woman, someone bites her left breast. There is a huge bite — hole — there. What is this hideous sexual imagery that keeps emerging from my being?

— July 8, 1975

How much I wish I could have been that warm person I see I can be now. I want to run back over yesterday and yell and scream and redo all that coldness I thought I was — those days I lost in icy coldness — and go back and show all the love that got lost in desperation. My chest caves in — the ocean — the icy waves. I cringe, desperately looking for love words. How sad, those people who cannot know that warmth is human. No warmth, no love.

— August 6, 1975

The emotional upheavals seem unmanageable. Serenity first. Turn life over to Higher Power for my own lesson learning. Always blamed the darkness on the food. Now, I see it is the attitude within me.

— March 16, 1976

Must remember to calm my emotions before acting.

— March 18, 1976

I want to do everything for everyone at once. Intense rage. I can't make decisions. Why choose one thing over another?

In my dream last night there was Sue's boyfriend. There was something bad and evil about him. They had a child so I took to caring for this baby. Strapped to my front chest, he laid snug and warm and safe from her. Blissfully sleeping, loved, nourished, we traveled through harm and yet no one, nothing could harm him. I loved him and protected him and he knew it and slept. I can still feel the warmth of his little body — snug. He knew he was safe and would not be harmed. Even as I knew we had to jump into the river to avoid danger, the baby was part of me and safe. I would protect it.

As he grew I took joy in watching his little mistakes, in seeing him learn and grow.

I journey back through childhood. Emotionally, I feel that old depression welling up inside my chest. But this time I perceive its extensions outward. I move inside the pain inside my chest and experience how it perceives the world. The world outside looks dark, confused. I try to move, to act — but I can move out into the world no farther than a few feet. I hit a wall and tumble backwards inside myself, tumbling, falling into the pit that is the pain inside my chest.

The paralysis unfolds. I see how it operates. If I can break through the wall that catches my movements and sends them back to me, I would be free. The wall — a construct in consciousness. It can be broken. It is being broken. Make a decision and act! Who cares if it is wrong?

When I was a child I was told what to do. I was not taught to rely on my own inner resources, on my own decisions. I was afraid to do for myself because I feared doing the wrong thing.

But now I see there is no right or wrong. The way lies only in the way I choose, and the mistakes I make, and the learning and growing I joyously do. Living is the process of exploring what one's own capacities are. Living is discovery.

– September 10, 1976

Now I see why I've felt so much hate. There was little expression of love in my family and I, being a sensitive child, inverted to rage and isolation. But feeling those lines open now, and communication occurs even now between my parents and me, and the feeling that they are there for me, when my father said, "Wake me if you want to eat, and talk to me."

– October 11, 1976

Feeling my caring — the nakedness and vulnerability of exposing the truth, being disliked and rebuffed and the awful feeling of being rejected rather than embraced for my love.

And then the fear of there being, if not a personal rejection, then a cosmic one, in which all of the sudden my perceptions will be proved wrong by the universe and there will exist a huge emptiness — a large, laughing, cosmic emptiness in which the largest and greatest force of all will reject us both — with nothing to say, nothing to exchange, no connectedness at all — and I will stand in shame, not only a self-condemnation but a condemnation from the universe itself, that all of my perceptions will prove to be lies.

— October 12, 1976

New found love of women. Dream last night of my being female. Anger at being the one expected to inspire a man's creativity, not the creative one. And then switch to female with child and the love and beauty of the event. I am not worthwhile unless I am as a man. Perhaps I shall go over to female side and respect femaleness for a while.

— November 1, 1976

No longer groping, I have strength. In the search amongst weeds, I cut those threads from me that hang unwanted and uncared for. I will not waste another moment of unwanted activity. There is no time for lies. The heart must follow and must guide, too, the mind and hand. No longer shall "should" dominate. Rather, "would" and "will" emanating from true desire.

— February, 1977

Grateful for seeing negativity.
Get myself out of me!
Make phone calls — when I feel negative, see how someone else is!

— March 4, 1977

Tenseness in throat. Loneliness, want to eat. Ate my breakfast for tomorrow. Feeling separate. I am all alone. Boyfriend? Jealous of Ellen and Ed. I am powerless over food — for today. Abstinence is the most important thing in my life. With it I can feel the pain and thus can handle it! Turn over to sponsor my food plan for tomorrow:
<u>*Lunch*</u>*: 1 green pepper*
1 cup zucchini
1 egg, 1 oz. Muenster
<u>*Dinner*</u>*: 1/2 chicken*
2 cup salad
1 cup zucchini

Binged!

— July 17, 1977

91

Sad and lonely over men. Want to eat but will choose to feel the pain, let it rise.

Binged!

— July 27, 1977

Loneliness again — food thoughts all day.
I'm judging myself. What's wrong with me that I am not out with someone?
Do I really want to be? Does it matter, really?
How can I work with it?

— August 3, 1977

Binged all night
Pain in heart and throat this morning. Upset about Chris and his girlfriend. I want a lover.

Dream:
Feel lonely and rejected. A couple with baby walks behind me. I am alone and I don't talk to them. In grandmother's house with sister, locking doors, afraid of people breaking in — fear of men.

Woke up depressed, angry.

— August 21, 1977

Dream:
Bruce asks our group what the biggest problem we are working on. I am very ashamed of mine and do want to say it. That I have been assaulted many times by men!

— September 4, 1977

Angry at Bruce for not calling me when I need him. Why doesn't he call? Like Steve, not being there when I need him! I suck them in because I need, demand their love, to be helped out of my desperation, rage, confusion. The only way I could get love was to manipulate for poor me.

I deserve to be loved for the actual me and I deserve to love.

— September 7, 1977

Need to work on letting my father touch me emotionally.

— October 16, 1977

Today I see how clearly I confuse my feeling of anger with compulsions — need to eat immediately. I wonder how many times my binges have been the result of angry feelings. How much rage and anger has not been dealt with because of powerless urge to eat.

— January 7, 1978

When my tiny, helpless infant is hungry and does not get fed, he gets very angry. Anger is his way of being heard, of making himself known, of feeling as if he has some control over his environment.

When we change my 2 1/2 year old son's diaper in spite of his attempts to prevent us from doing so, he also gets very angry. This is his way of maintaining his sense of identity, asserting his desires, making his needs known.

As I study my sons' anger, I realize that anger is one way we attempt to assert our individuality in this world. If we come from a background in which our individuality has been "swallowed," as in an eating disorder, it is not surprising that many of us feel rage when we begin to heal. After denying ourselves — keeping our feelings inside, our needs inside, perhaps not even knowing who we are — when we begin to let ourselves open up, a gush of anger rushes forth: anger at not getting needs met, anger at not being heard. Anger is the first way we know to assert our power. Until we know what we want, until we know who we are, until more constructive ways are learned, the only way we have to assert our power is through anger. That is okay. It is necessary. It is an important stage through which to pass.

I pounded pillows and threw bottles. That was my infantile phase. Then I realized I needed to direct that energy more constructively. As I started to find ways to assert myself, feel more in control of me, know my needs and get them met, my anger subsided.

I still had to learn how to handle my anger. It became an easy way out. It became too familiar, a way to block my growth. My frequent anger became a way of not having to go deeper, a way of not having to find my way of walking in the world.

Justified anger: temper tantrums at not being given my way. Resentful of my job for treating me unjustly — not enough pay and too long hours. What are the alternatives to tantrums and resentments?
God, what would you have me do?
Take positive action to find work elsewhere.

— January 8, 1978

When we were little children perhaps we were punished for being angry, or disapproved of, or yelled back at — most likely we weren't taught how to handle anger. What I usually experienced was: someone yells, another yells back; or someone yells, another runs away. No one seems to understand how to relate to anger constructively. I like dialoguing with my anger. I like to find solutions. I very much dislike venting anger and going nowhere with it. As little children our anger was probably rarely taken seriously, so we grew up not taking our own anger seriously. This is unfortunate, because as an adult I've come to learn my anger usually has something important to tell me. It is usually an indication that a real need is not being met, or that I am expecting too much from myself. If I work with my anger constructively, I'm challenged to find a way to listen to the message behind the anger.

When my son gets angry, it is usually because his father and I have neglected his needs. Because of this, we try to meet his needs as much as possible — because we want him to learn his needs are important. It could get pretty frustrating as a child to have one's needs constantly ignored. I would think that one would begin to harbor a lot of anger and grow up feeling angry all the time "for no good reason." How many of us adult addicts walk around feeling our needs just aren't as important as another's? We repress our anger because we believe "anger" is a nuisance of an emotion and only gets us in trouble. At one time it probably did get us in trouble. However, today, not to express our anger will get us into worse trouble. It is vital we learn to work with our anger constructively. It is vital for our health and the health of those with whom we live. We owe it to ourselves and to others to listen to the message our anger relays.

(A great book on the subject is *Dr. Weisinger's Anger Work-Out* by Hendrie Weisinger, Ph.D.)

Fear of failure: I set up the condition of having to have it done in a month. Maybe this is not God's will. I programmed a good pressure cooker with a good chance of failing or bingeing.

– February 21, 1978

Want to change food plan. Overeat — extra farmer cheese.
Dinner — large salad, no dressing and part of tomorrow's chicken, extra squash.
In a lot of pain — emotional. Feel despair of why be in the "now" with no dreams and no goals, just emptiness. Grab for goals to fill in the emptiness. Always looking to where I'm going. Put me in the "now" with no goals, no desires pushing me on and I feel desperate, sad, lonely. What for, what's the use? I remember waking today feeling the emptiness.

– March 7, 1978

Binged.

Fear of making mistakes.
Working too hard, not able to take care of food.
See, here I am, the old Jane, worthless, can do nothing but eat.

Of course, I'm not suited for success. If I hadn't binged I would have been success-ful of sorts. This way, I could prove I am a constant failure and not worthy of earning the life of a healthy, happy, beautiful human being.

It's exciting! I'm not going to give into those feelings — focus my identity on creating a successful, beautiful person!

– July 5, 1978

Fear — frightened of being lonely, alone, without love and intimacy.

God — please remove my fear of being alone. Afraid of being alone without any friends. Dear God, remove this fear and let me feel the love and your presence and guide me to act and relate to my true Self. Perhaps I am to develop deeper friend-ships with more people.

– June 7, 1979

Softly I walk
Beyond the evening
Into the cool lake place
blue and silver hue
pinkness gathering clouds
lightly
rising
into
joy

Twirls of threads-golden
woven into fragrant softness
My inner arms stretch wide
further than before
not afraid
to feel.

– August, 1979

IN SUMMARY

Happiness can never come from how one eats. It can only come from how one feels inside.

Exercise your observer. You are not the same as your emotions.
Keep a diary of your feelings.

Accept all of your feelings non-judgmentally.

In order to effectively manage your emotions you must
1) Realize you alone are responsible for your emotions
2) Magnify your observer

Some tools for working with feelings are:
1) Discuss your feelings with others
2) Dialogue
3) Release negative emotions
4) Channel life-energy
5) Channel light-fire

A lot of sadness. I want to feel close to myself all of the time, not just when I'm in the country or at an OA meeting. Hugging all the time, because everyone is beautiful. Desperately needing and holding on to those meetings for inner warmth, and if I'm deprived I'm in a panic. No, Jane — darling, I love you, feel the warmth from the light. Know that the sun shines from deep inside to warm the skin from the inside out.

There is loneliness and fear. It is an illusion that separates me. It is inner love and warmth that I want, not food.

– August 13, 1976

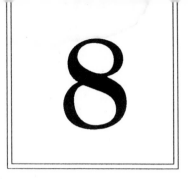

Loving and Forgiving Myself
and Others

My Attitude Toward My Body. My Attitude Toward My Bingeing.
My Attitude Toward My Weaknesses. My Attitude Toward Other People's Bodies.
My Attitude Toward Other People's Weaknesses. Support Networks.
No Fear Now.

Need to bring forth beauty and love in small matters. Heart opens and I see the flower
that is there if I allow it to blossom.

– April 6, 1977

If I had to name the single most important thing I did for my recovery from compulsive eating, I would say it was the ongoing process of loving and forgiving myself. If you were a mother with a sick child, would you hate it because it was sick? Or would you love and care for it until it got better?

LOVE HEALS

This simple truth works in all areas of life, whether it is the hate you feel for another, for yourself, for something you've done or for a part of your body.

Most of us are afraid that if we accept our overweight, we will lose our motivation to change. I was afraid to love myself fat. I was afraid to love my bingeing. I was afraid that if I loved myself I would lose my motivation to lose weight and stop bingeing. But I found the contrary to be true. When I binged, the shame fed my low self-esteem. I felt unworthy of even attempting to change my life for the better. As I started forgiving myself, the guilt and shame lessened. As I forgave myself, I became more self-confident and, as I became more self-confident, I became stronger. Each time I forgave myself, my self-esteem increased. As I felt worthier, I felt better able to make changes, to do the things necessary to replace the bingeing with constructive action.

The areas of my life that were most in need of change were:
1. My attitude towards my body.
2. My attitude towards my bingeing.
3. My attitude towards my weaknesses.
4. My attitude towards other people's bodies.
5. My attitude towards other people's weaknesses.

Bruce comments on my sexy dress. I feel intensely ashamed, awkward about my body. Jane, what a fool you are, why didn't you wear something else? I hate my big breasts and hips, feel awkward.

– August 21, 1977

What woman doesn't know what it feels like to hate at least some part of her body? We all strive for that ideal thin body — the one seen in magazine ads and television commercials.

Society's emphasis on being thin will only change as each of us individually makes the change within ourself. We must become aware of our brainwashing. Watch the commercials on television with an objective eye. Look at the magazine ads. What about most of our Hollywood stars? For the most part, they have the same type of body, don't they? The same is true of the mannequins in our department stores. Everywhere you look, you are being told that you do not fit in unless you have that certain look. Now, take a good look at the women you work with, the women on the street, the women in supermarkets or any other public place. Watch them closely. How many of them actually look the way they are "supposed to"? Not very many. Compare yourself to them. Are you really that different?

We must come to realize our worth is not dependent solely on how we look. Our personal sense of identity, rather, must be determined by what we think, feel and do. In this society, we are raised to believe that our appearance determines our worth. Men have much more of themselves identified with what they do. We, as women, need to start changing this.

EXERCISE

Make a list of the activities you enjoy doing, the activities you would like to do if you had more time and energy. Post that list in a prominent place in your home. When you begin to obsess about your looks, about what you ate, about dieting, go to your list and choose an activity that would be fun to do instead — and do it. You need to take the energy that is consumed by obsessive thinking and put it into pleasurable activities. Soon, your new energy direction will become habit. Your self-confidence will increase. Your attitude towards yourself and your body will change. Your body will become a tool through which to enjoy life's pleasures.

Learn how to send love to me first and then turn outward to give that love to others.
— June 1, 1979

I am bringing healing energy into the areas of my body that I dislike — my thighs, hips, stomach, breasts, calves.
— June 2, 1979

Send love messages to your body. Work on changing your body image.

Dress comfortably. Throw away or store all clothes that are too small or uncomfortable to wear. It is very difficult to love a body that is being pinched by waistbands that are too small or is afraid to move for fear of popping a button. When you wear clothes that fit loosely, your body will begin to breathe and move freely.

Treat yourself to a weekly or monthly massage. This does wonders for releasing stress and discomfort. It is very difficult to love a body that is tense and tight. Find a masseur/masseuse with whom you feel comfortable. You should feel as if love is being channeled from him/her to you through touch. This is very important because your body will respond to the love that is channeled. You, in turn, will learn to channel love to your body more quickly.

Explore body awareness techniques such as Alexander, Feldenkrais, Rolfing, Hellerwork, Yoga, Tai Chi, etc. (Check the resource list on pages 123-128 for specific addresses and telephone numbers.) It is important to learn how to move with the flow of energy — moving with yourself, not against yourself. Many overweight or obsessive people have learned to hold themselves in self-defeating ways. The body will learn to adopt negative postures in alignment with negative feelings. It then tends to "lock in" these feelings, physically making them very resistant to change and causing unnecessary tension and low energy states. Body/mind is a union — two sides of the same coin. Liberate your body from self defeating postures and habits of movement, and you will liberate your mind.

Desire to be beautiful as expression of love, as a mirror of inner beauty, radiance and love. Want to dress sexually. Special project: change self-image to express radiance.

    I used to dress to protest.
    I do not dress to attract.
    I dress to be accepted, to find security with a group.
    I dress with an "I don't care" message.
    How can I flatter and enhance instead of hide my body?

                                              – July 2, 1979

I do not know my reproduction system. Rituals and rites of sexuality growing into consciousness, in celebration. I am a circle. I am a cycle. I am now in my ovary, my fallopian tube, my uterus, my vaginal canal. And every month I must acknowledge the change in my body. I must acknowledge and celebrate that part of me that is female.

Trying to ignore its screams for acknowledgment – splitting me. I try to hide my eyes so as not to see and be the blood.

Women, instead of pretending we are not, we must celebrate it!

                                            – March 25, 1979

EXERCISE

    Here is an excellent body awareness exercise:

1.   Begin by channeling life-energy, as directed, up through Step 3 of the basic life-energy exercise on page 49.

2.   Intensify the energy in specific areas of your body. Do this very slowly. Intensify the energy in your feet, legs, hips and pelvic bowl, stomach and digestive tract, heart, lungs, shoulders, neck, face, head, and hair. Note your reactions to the areas of your body you are traveling in. Think of intensifying the energy in the areas that are the most uncomfortable. Think of this energy as your "love" energy.

3.   If you encounter any particularly difficult areas, (such as "darkness" or pain) think of intensifying the "fire" aspect of the energy to burn or consume obstacles to well-being.

When I first did this, I was unable to move into my pelvic area and thighs. It was as if there was a wall preventing me from entering those spaces. As I continued this exercise I thought of amplifying the energy in that area, and eventually I was able to enter. At first I felt disgusted but slowly, as I continued to amplify the energy and send feelings of love, my pelvic area opened to the love and began to absorb the light.

This exercise works, but it is difficult. Because your negative feelings and sensations may be new to you and feel overwhelming, you may want to give up. Don't. It might be a good idea to work with a counselor, someone who can help you understand particularly difficult sensations or emotions that might arise. If you have someone to help you, great. If not, do a little every day, not more than you feel you can handle on your own. Those little bits add up. One day you will wake up and say, "Hey, I like myself." What a good feeling that is.

EXERCISE

One way to begin loving your body is to talk to it and listen to what it has to say. Communicating with others is one way we express our caring. Why shouldn't we do the same with our bodies? The "dialogue" tool has been a wonderful way of discovering my body's needs.

1. Dialogue with your body when you want to binge. Start out with the question, "Why do you want to binge?"

2. Dialogue with your body while you are bingeing.

3. Dialogue with a part of your body that is in chronic pain.

4. Dialogue with your body as a whole.

5. Dialogue with your fat. Ask it what it wants to tell you about itself, why it exists, what function it has in your life.

6. Dialogue with the parts of you that you dislike the most.

Dialogue With Body (1974)

J(ane) - Body, why am I stuffing you with food right now?
B(ody) - You don't want to feel.

J - What don't I want to feel?

B - Your excitement. It has no place to go.

J - I am very excited. I just wrote that dialogue with Philip and realized how I set the situation up to alienate him from me and for me to be angry at him.

B - I know. I wrote it with pen in hand.

J - Oh, cut it out.

B - Well, stop hurting me. It wasn't my fault that you had an understanding. I'm getting pretty pissed off that every time you have an insight you take it out on me. It's beginning to really bug the hell out of me. Why do you do it?

J - I asked you first.

B - You tell me. I don't have a mind.

J - Well — No, I need your insights. I've just had some. I'm scared.

B - Good start. You are scared. What of?

J - Well, I don't know what's going to happen to me with all this new knowledge. I've changed and who am I?

B - I don't know who you are, but I'm still the same and I still don't like being stuffed with food.

J - I feel sick. Why doesn't Philip call so I can tell him that I'm sorry for creating an ugly situation and tell him what I've discovered. Oh, I feel sick. My stomach is jumping.

B - After all that cheese and ice-cream you should feel sick.

J - I'll vomit it up.

B - Sure. Old habits, old habits.

J - Come on. God, I don't know what to do.

B - Listen to some music.

Dialogue with Heart (1974)

J(ane) - Heart, why are you in tension and pain?

H(eart) - I ache for all the people who cannot love.

J - But I always thought that the ache was mine.

H - No, the ache is mine only. Don't confuse it with yourself.

J - Oh heart, why am I crying now?

H - You feel so much, Jane, all the sensations that come into you, you mistake for yourself. As they go through you —

J - Well, what about the business with Philip?

H - You pick up his hurt so strongly and mistake it for your own. You are afraid to acknowledge this, because it changes your identity. Then you cannot be the martyr of all others' pain. You hold the pain of the world on your chest and you pride yourself in it.

Dialogue with Body (1974)

J(ane) - Your capacity for pleasure is small. You are a royal pain in the ass. You prevent me from doing what I want to do. There is no controlling you. When I'm welding, you're eating. When I'm dancing, you are fat. When I'm making sculpture you are pacing. You need sugar out of nowhere. You feel pained in the chest or throat.

B(ody) - You don't take care of me. You hate me.

J - How can I help but hate you when you always get in my way.

B - But now I'm not fat.

J - Yeah, but you still go numb and cause me discomfort, going dizzy or paralyzed or pained, striking me down.

B - I'm better now because you're caring for me more. You are more inside me. You have more respect for me. I remember when you got your haircut. I was so pleased. You cared enough for me to go to a professional hairdresser.

J - But why were you so opposed to me, so against everything I did?

B - Because you hated me.

J - I would have liked you if you were prettier.

B - See. Always caring for the superficial. You wanted me to serve your image of the perfect dancer's body. You never saw who I was and cared for me. I wasn't Margot Fonteyn's body. I was Jane's. So I rebelled against you.

J - When did it begin?

B- Maybe when you were eleven and cried because you didn't want to grow old, how disrespectful of my process.

J - How absurd.

B - Don't laugh.

J - You are a devil.

B - You bet. You better love me!

J - Okay. I succumb. Where do I begin? I know, care about your health and diet. I guess when you act up it's because you are angry.

B - Maybe.

J - You are sly.

B - Look, dear. When I act up, I'm just asserting myself.

J - How do I conquer you?

B - Not by conquering, by caring.

J - Okay. Next time your right side goes numb I'll caress it, talk to it, ask it what's the matter.

B - I sense a cynicism.

J - Yes, I'm a bit disgusted.

B - Because you cannot be without me and you are finally admitting it.

J - Why do I hate you so much?

B - Because I am a devil. I've always been one.

J - You make me sick, puke! You make me want to puke. You rebellious little monster. I hate your guts. Get out of my life.

B - I can't. I am your life. But you can get out of me.

J - I'm working at it, believe me. I'd love to astral project!

B - You know those motives are perverse and you can't solve anything by running away.

J - Yeah. I'm always trying to run away. Okay, you do give me some pleasure. Maybe I can list the things I love about you.
I love your hands.
I love the energy I feel in my skin and head, the energy rushing through me.
I love the feeling of my lungs expanding and dilating and the air going through me.
I love my imagination.
I love when P. touches my head and neck.
I love massages and long hot baths.
I love to feel you move and do things I never imagined you'd do when dancing.

B - It seems to me you love a lot about me.

J - Yes.

B - Please love more.

J - I will make a list of things I want to love.

B - Okay.

J - I want to love the feel of food enter into me, the feel of my muscles moving as I walk. I want to love the feel of caressing pain, of easing tension. I want to love the tension so that I might alleviate it. I want to love the highs and not be so afraid of them.

The way I began expressing love was through forgiveness. I learned to forgive my imperfections and I forgave myself every time I binged! No joke. The next time you binge say to yourself:

"I have binged and I want to hate myself for it. I want to feel ashamed. I want to hide my head in the sand, beat myself up, kill myself. But I will not do any of those things. Instead, I will acknowledge that I am human and that I have a weakness. My weakness is food, but I am working to get stronger. One of the things I am doing is forgiving myself for my imperfections. Therefore, I will forgive myself right here, right now. I will learn from this experience. I will use it as a challenge to grow."

I then ask myself the following questions: What events preceded the binge? What was I feeling? Was there another way to deal with this incident or with my feelings? What could I have done?

After I had answered these questions I was sure to find something to do that gave me pleasure. I remember my mandala drawing phase. I loved drawing the circles and repetitive, symmetric designs over and over again. It occupied my hands and mind and helped center me. Try to find something to do that is soothing and centering — perhaps sewing, quilting, knitting, ceramics or playing a musical instrument.

As I binged less, I discovered things about myself that appalled me. I discovered I was arrogant. I made mistakes. I was too critical of others. I was afraid of people. I could say stupid things. Needless to say, I became more and more unhappy with who I was.

One of the functions of bingeing, I have found, is to protect us from an awareness of some of the real symptoms of our low self-esteem. Somehow it is easier to hate ourselves for bingeing than to hate ourselves for failing, making mistakes, saying stupid things, being afraid and judging others.

With this in mind, be forewarned. Do not expect a bed of roses when you stop bingeing. Do not expect to love yourself because you no longer have a problem with food. Do expect, however, to discover things about yourself that could be painful. But, if you remember to forgive your imperfections, you will be able to transform those behavior traits as well.

Remember: You are not alone. No one can claim perfection. Perfection does not exist except in our imaginations.

EXERCISE

At night, before you go to sleep, make a journal entry. Divide a clean sheet of paper into two parts. On the left, list all your faults. Think of everything you did, said and felt that day. What were you unhappy with? Did you get angry with someone unnecessarily? Did you make an error on the job? Did you say something you regretted? What would you like to improve? After you have completed the list, fully forgive yourself everything. Love yourself unconditionally. *Know that you are all right exactly the way you are today!* When you have accepted and forgiven yourself — your thoughts, feelings and deeds — write down on the other side of the paper what you would like to improve. It is important to know that it is possible to accept yourself unconditionally while improving yourself at the same time.

EXERCISE

Get completely relaxed, sitting or lying down.

1. Move with your awareness to a place 6" above the top of your head. We will call this your "Upper Room." It is the home of your Self or your personal Higher Power. This is the place where you can go in awareness anytime you wish to contact the part of you that is already enlightened. This place is glowing, radiant and full of unconditional love.

2. Experience what happens as you think of radiant awareness flowing down from the Upper Room into your brain, gathering and uplifting your own mental awareness, sending love and radiance into your thoughts and mental processes, harmonizing them with the radiant awareness of unobstructed consciousness.

3. Think of radiant awareness flowing down into the neurons of your brain and neural pathways of your body, gathering and enlightening your sensory awareness. This is the part of you that is responsible for how you perceive or "sense" the world — your attitudes and perceptions. Experience what happens as this part of you is harmonized with the love and radiance that comes from Self.

4. Now, think of radiant awareness flowing down into your heart and circulatory system, gathering and enlightening your feeling awareness. Experience what happens as your emotional nature is harmonized with the radiant love.

5.   Sit still, experiencing radiant awareness uplifting and enlightening all three aspects of your personality — your knowing, sensory and emotional natures.

6.   Now move back into the spaces of your Upper Room. Remember, this is the place where you can go to best contact your actual Self. The size of this Self is relative to how you wish to perceive it. For this exercise, think of it becoming a size just a bit larger than that of your physical body and experience as you comfortably snuggle inside this Being of Light. Experience the radiance and love emanating from it. Open yourself to allow this radiance and love to pour into you — every bit of you — your physical self, as well as your knowing, sensory and feeling self. Let all self-hatred, fear, and guilt be lovingly scooped up by this radiant Being and pulled out of the spaces of your body. Think of all the spaces of your body opening to release the negativity, the conditioning. Experience what happens as unconditional love surrounds you — all of you — and pours into every part of you.

7.   Be still, absorbing this love and radiance. Quietly assimilate the essence pouring into you from this grand, powerful, and all-loving Being. This is your true Self sending unconditional love to your splintered and hurting selves. This is healing essence.

If you are self-critical, you are probably also critical of others.

Do you look at others and see them as thin or fat? I bet you do. If you do, you have a filter in your mind that is responsible for perceiving the world (and yourself in the world) as either thin or fat. You need to change this filter. It is that simple.

EXERCISE

The goal here will be to replace that filter with one that is more appropriate for becoming binge-free. This new filter will not see people as fat or thin. Instead, it will see people's bodies as a variety of interesting forms and shapes. Begin by becoming observant of the objects in your environment and in nature. Notice, without judgment, the variety of form that surrounds you. Notice the many shapes and sizes of trees, flowers, and animals. Now try to view each human body in the same way — notice its particular curves, and the way it moves through space. Note its particular beauty. As you get in the habit of doing this, you will discover that the way people are shaped can be a form of aesthetic pleasure. All shapes and forms can be pleasing if you choose to look at them that way.

Just very aware all day of the thoughts that run between me and the external environment, as I was with Ginny and Tommy and could hear my head judging, weighing every comment they made, seeing if they met up to standards I set. Extremely aware of my cautiousness and the extent to which my negative thoughts weigh. No one fits with that running ideal!

— October 26, 1974

A counselor once told me something that changed my life. He said, "You are too critical. You need to see the good that is in everyone." The words stung. I knew he was telling the truth.

I began watching my thoughts when I was with others, and I saw how I automatically started criticizing people. I never seemed to see the good in anybody. To change this way of thinking, I began making mental notes of any good qualities, no matter how small they seemed to be. I worked at forgiving others as I tried to forgive myself.

The following example, although extreme, powerfully illustrates how the way we perceive others can affect the way we live our lives. About twelve years ago, a strange man broke into my apartment and attempted to rape me. My first reaction was to kill. Who wouldn't feel this way? My counselor suggested I forgive this man. "You are asking the impossible," I said.

"Think of him as being a victim of his own upbringing. Maybe he was terribly abused as a child. Maybe he suffers a pain so deep nothing you have ever felt can come close to it. Perhaps his attack on you was the only way he knew to ask for help."

I pondered these words for a long time. I then sat down in quiet reflection and brought his terrible image into my mind. I fought my desire to kill and, instead, allowed love energy to flow from me to him. I felt an incredible release within my own spaces. I was free. I wept for him and for myself and for all those who are victims of their own self-hatred. Was he really that different from me? I abused myself with food. He abused others. All we both really wanted or needed was love. He eventually took his own life. I knew mine would be saved.

February, 1984

Dear Support Group Members,

I never liked group situations. A large part of me still doesn't, and yet I love this group and how it makes me feel.

In the beginning, usually before we start, I feel uncomfortable. If I see two or three people together, laughing, I feel left out. If someone is getting a lot of attention from other members of the group, I feel jealous and competitive. I want to yell out, "Why aren't you giving me that attention!" For a split second fear overwhelms me. I feel rejected, left out, desperate. They like her better than me. I'm quiet, trying to find a way out of this dilemma, trying hard to find a way to get some attention, to feel acknowledged. And then it is as if everyone conspires against me. EVERY-ONE! I turn to my right, trying to catch the eye of a familiar face, but there is no response. She does not see me. I am invisible. She looks right through me. Every-one is looking through me.

But why? What is this about? How can I be recovered when parts of me still need so much? How can I be recovered and still feel so helpless, rejected, worthless?

The question of "recovery" seems to be a major one for all of us. If we are ill we want to know what we can look forward to. How much hope can we realisti-cally have? How much recovery is possible? Will we be obsessed with food and our bodies our entire lives? Will we be slaves to support groups, food plans, psychother-apy, our whole lives? Will we ever be able to eat and be like "normal people?" People have asked me, how do you know you are recovered? What does it feel like?

Although my original intention in coming to this support group was to give support, in the process I am finding out why, when I was bulimic, I stayed so isolated. Why should anyone want to face these threatening feelings? It was easier to stay home alone eating, much safer just to stay away from groups, and not feel threatened by others. In becoming aware of these feelings, I have discovered parts of me that need healing. I am surprised to find out there are parts of me that still feel lonely and are in need of love. But the difference between being bulimic and being recovered is that I no longer turn to food to fill that need for love; I no longer confuse those parts of me with the whole me; and I have other ways to deal with those uncomfortable feelings.

Why is it, despite these uncomfortable feelings, when our support group ends, I feel filled with so much love, I hate to leave? Why is it I have trouble sleeping, thinking about all the things we shared with one another? The love I feel for every-one is just as real a part of me as the fear .

My recovery has been an ongoing process of learning how to look at the ugly parts of myself. I have had to be as honest with others as I've had to be with myself. I've also learned to know that the ugly parts of me were never the whole me, that there has been and always will be a beautiful side of me that has such a capacity for love, no fear or anger or loneliness can match that magnitude and wealth.

I am recovered because food no longer takes the place of looking deep within my psyche.

I am recovered because I am not afraid to admit to myself or to those I love that I am not perfect.

I am recovered because I have found a way to work with my imperfections so that I can change them and grow.

I am recovered because I choose to act from the positive parts of me, not the negative.

The next step will be to channel love to the parts of me that are still hurting. Only when they feel loved will they stop feeling threatened by you. And only then will I be able to come to the group and feel as good in the beginning as I do at the end.

A support network should provide unconditional support. The members of the network say to one another, "I accept all parts of you and your feelings unconditionally. I allow you to grow, change, be who you are without expectation." It is easy to wish our parents and siblings had been this way. It is easy to wish our spouses felt this way about us, or us about them. But to wish this is a fruitless activity. In order to learn to love and accept ourselves we need to find people who support us in this way. We need to find people who will mirror back to us the unconditional love we need to feel for ourselves.

OA was my first support network. The people there accepted every part of me, including the part of me that binged. For the first time in my life I felt understood and completely accepted. I had also found a group of people who worked with life-energy; that was my second support group.*

Both these groups taught me to see myself as God saw me — a beautiful creation put on this earth to be the best that I could be, to forgive myself my faults and weaknesses, to accept my frailties and my imperfections. I came to know that

---

* Overeater's Anonymous has the greatest number of support groups. More and more hospitals are also opening eating disorder inpatient and outpatient clinics. ANAD is another organization that has groups in many major cities in the U.S. See the resource list on pages 123-128 for information on a number of potential support networks.

God loved me just as I was and forgave me my wrongs. Because I saw this mirrored in the faces of the beautiful people who could also accept and forgive me, I began to accept myself, to forgive myself and to flourish.

How far back can I trace my lack of nourishment? It goes way back, as far back as the whispering memory of cells and organs will take me. Only after many years of emptiness, emotional starvation, frustration, am I now free to find the fulfillment that only inner nourishment can provide.

Life is too beautiful for us not to know that somehow, somewhere we can find and claim that beauty for ourselves. There is always something that will touch our hearts, maybe for but a brief moment — a tree as it blossoms in spring, the fresh scent of country, the sounds of birds, perhaps its in another's love — these things remind us that life is not for struggle, but is rather for deep contentment, exalted love, profound peace. I believe this is what a baby knows, a baby who is nourished, well loved, protected.

At fifteen I ate compulsively and screamed hysterically, "Why can't I stop? Please mother, I want to die!" How many children know this feeling? Why? What are they missing? I do not believe it is merely the "stresses" of modern life. No, I believe it is a malfunction of caring. Somewhere along the way the ability to love had been lost. Love is life's sustenance. Without it, we bend at every turn. With it we can stand firm and fight the little stresses of each day.

I was a compulsive eater. I awoke depressed, stayed depressed, went to sleep depressed. I found my solace in the deadening of my pain. I was stubborn. I was irrational. I was full of hate; I knew no other way. But you see, now I can go back. I can fill that emptiness from within. As a child I was dependent upon mother, and mother didn't do it. As an adult I can let the Divine Mother within fill me until there is no more room. With that I can change the destiny of my life.

As I hold a memory still — a point of time — and feel into the pain, the emptiness, I ask true Self to fill that memory with abundant love. Sometimes I must hold it still for many many minutes. So much defensiveness has been built around that pain, it takes much patience before I can feel the softening and opening to the love that is my true birthright. When I feel the pain leave, when the past brightens, I know then that I have changed forever, and a portion of my future will unfold anew. The flood gates open and Mother gushes forth to nourish. I am supported in every thought, action, movement. Every moment is upheld. There will be no loss, for each move I make is connected with the movement of the universe. Where Self supports there is only abundance. I will be provided for because I walk in harmony with the universe. No fear now.

EXERCISE

1. Begin by channeling life-energy, as directed, up through Step 3 of the basic exercise on page 49.

2. Think back to a painful moment in childhood. Hold that memory in your mind and feel the pain now that you felt then. Let that moment be a still point in time. Think of sending forth a radiant, healing, loving energy. Bathe the experience in this luxurious light and allow yourself to forgive, experiencing newness in this moment, the essence of pain released.

IN SUMMARY

Love Heals

When we love, we become stronger — our self-esteem is increased. As our self-esteem increases, so does our ability to change and grow.

Accept yourself unconditionally — the way you are now.

Send love:
>To your body
>To your bingeing
>To your weaknesses
>To other people who have hurt and disappointed you

There is no way that I can progress spiritually with the continuation of binges and the chaotic, devastating results these moments bring. And if I continue to destroy myself spiritually I will ultimately destroy my whole self because I know that without spiritual work my life will be worthless.

— July 15, 1976

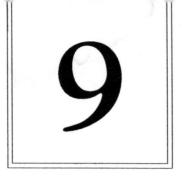

My Spiritual Awakening

The Spiritual Path to Freedom from Addiction.

One morning I awoke feeling very depressed. I had a bunch of chores to do — get my little boy off to the sitter's, breakfast dishes, laundry, sweeping — before sitting quietly down to write. But the pain of depression was persistent. I tried to ignore it. "I can't waste my time with this pain," I tried to tell myself, hoping it would go away. Anyone who's felt it knows how insidious and persistent depression can be; it invades every aspect of one's life with feelings of hopelessness, despair, and desolation. This time was no different. I couldn't get rid of it.

I finally reconciled myself to the fact that this was going to be one of those mornings when no work got done. I had to tend to these feelings if I was going to be able to function in any capacity at all. With diary and pen in hand, I sat quietly in deep solitude. I cried a little, and then my hand began to write. I asked my first question, the question I always begin with when I start one of these dialogues, "Who are you? What do you want from me? Why are you causing me this pain?" I saw some bent and broken beings crouched in pain, and then the answers began to come. "You have been ignoring us," they said. "Who are you?" I asked again. "We are the part of you that connects with spirit."

It was true. I had been ignoring my spirit. I had been so busy trying to get ahead, take care of a child, start a business and write a book, that I had stopped allocating any of my time to meditation, reflection and personal exploration.

As I continued to dialogue, I was given a new perspective on the activities I was performing in my outer life and was taken to a special place — a spiritual place of learning.

When I was through with this special dialogue and journey and opened my eyes, not only was my depression gone, but I felt especially full of love for life. My energy was revitalized, and I felt rich in new understanding of what I was doing and where I was going with my work.

The story of my spiritual awakening began over fourteen years ago. One day, after a Rolfing session, while riding a New York subway, I was struck by an overwhelming feeling that I and everything I could see from my vantage point were ONE. I was literally lifted into an "altered" state of consciousness. I felt at once all powerful and humbled. I was larger than life, as if the sense of who I was radiated outward to encompass all that surrounded me. I was in the everpresent NOW. I was at peace.

As expected, this powerful experience became less and less intense as the weeks went by but its essence remained in me as a reminder that there was and always will be a world beyond the one in which we ordinarily function.

Because of my addiction I was forced to find a way of functioning from this spiritual world on a daily basis. What I found was the deep place within. From this place I can feel the meaning of my existence, the reason for being here. I can contact the deep earth and feel a part of the universe. Yes, there are many stars, many grains of sand, many leaves, many countless cells — but each one has its place and is indispensable to the whole. From this deep place I feel connected, not alone, a part of the grand scheme of things.

And from this deep place I can feel the rightness of being where I now am, no escaping the perfectness of my existence in the way it is unfolding. If I go too long without contacting the deep place within, I begin to feel lost; life becomes meaningless and I start to despair. I must maintain contact with my Self because it is from that source that I am nourished and can grow.

Was my eating, indeed devouring, not a way I once tried to get that nourishment — a desperate searching for deep fulfillment; a seeking for deep satisfaction, for meaning behind the surface appearance of things? Devour, ingest — turn away from the outside world — turn within myself — ingest more, go deeper, escape from the meaningless activities out there — looking for peace, solace, hungering for safety and love.

Now, I search with my breath, my pen, my eyes and find that deep place — no need to eat to run from outer distraction. I can now go within and be nourished, essence pouring forth.

And where is my journey headed?

To help others transform the compulsive need to devour into a positive search for inner nourishment.

The structure that is making way for the new is the old life of diseased compulsion and the need to heal myself from my disease that has been completed. That structure is no longer needed and with that destruction there is new birth to levels unknown to me now. But the sorrow I felt tonight is a sorrow for old life patterns and images leaving forever — the old identities, Jane as compulsive eater giving way to Jane, new, not known yet, and the emptiness of old life gone. Perhaps despair will come upon me as "emptiness" is felt while awaiting the new to be born.

— February 17, 1980

Parting Words

My journey to freedom from bingeing was a long but exciting one. Although I no longer have an eating problem, I've grown to love the kind of exploration my problem once *demanded* I do. Today I continue to use these tools, not because I have to, but because I want to. The problems that I still have to deal with in the other areas of my life have become much more manageable as a result of that work.

The riches that are within enable me to live a life that to others must look rather boring. I do not need the "thrills" of artificially-produced excitement because my thrills are found within the pockets of my own psyche. The "high" I once derived from sugar, caffeine or diet pills is no longer desirable. "Emptiness" and "boredom" are no longer words in my personal vocabulary. Depression and anger are no longer emotions to be afraid of, but have become, instead, valued messages from my subconscious that action needs to be taken.

If I have been able to communicate one thing to you, I hope it has been this: **Compulsive eating is a symptom of things gone awry. It is a camouflaged, but accessible, communication to you from your subconscious.** Don't run from it! Listen to it. Let it tell you what it's saying. You can learn to value its function in your life if you work at deciphering the code.

As you do, you will begin to discover the excitement of making your own acquaintance — and the deep sense of fulfillment that comes from nurturing your most valued friend — you. Please don't let this opportunity pass. Nourish yourself — nurture yourself. Learn to stop dieting, stop bingeing, take risks and explore. It is your life. Don't let it pass you by.

RESOURCES

These listings do not imply an endorsement. The organizations mentioned are worth checking out, but as always — each of us has to decide for ourselves whether a given book, workshop or teacher truly serves our own needs.

Eating Disorder Organizations
(The following eating disorder organizations are non-profit and would appreciate your enclosing $1.00 to cover mailing costs.)

American Anorexia/Bulimia Association
(AA/BA)
133 Cedar Lane
Teaneck NJ 07666
(201) 836-1800

Anorexia Nervosa and Bulimia Foundation
Box 19855
Seattle WA 98109
(206) 322-6761

Anorexia Nervosa and Related Eating Disorders, Inc.
(ANRED)
Box 5102
Eugene OR 97405
(503) 344-1144

Bulimia Anorexia Self-Help (BASH)
6125 Clayton Ave., Suite 215
St. Louis MO 63139
(314) 567-4080 or (314) 991-BASH

Center for the Study of Anorexia and Bulimia
1 West 91st St.
New York NY 10024
(212) 595-3449

Foundation for Education about Eating Disorders
(FEED)
Box 34
Boring MD 21020
(301) 429-4918

National Anoriexia Aid Society, Inc.
(NAAS)
5796 Karl Road
Columbus OH 43229
(614) 436-1112

National Association to Aid Fat Americans, Inc.
(NAAFA)
P.O. Box 43
Bellerose NY 11426

National Association of Anorexia Nervosa and Associated Disorders
(ANAD)
Box 7
Highland Park IL 60035
(312) 831-3438

Overeaters Anonymous
World Service Office
2190 190th St.
Torrance CA 90504
(213) 775-2368

Bodywork, Meditation, Personal Growth and Health Organizations

Actualism
739 E. Pennsylvania, Suite D
Escondido CA 92026
(714) 741-7827

Training in life-energy work. Training centers in southern California and
New York City.

American Academy of Environmental Medicine
(formerly Society for Clinical Ecology)
Box 16106
Denver CO 80216

They will provide a list of physicans in a particular geographic area, information on environmental medicine and a list of educational publications. They ask for a S.A.S.E. and $2.40 to cover their costs.

The American Center of the Alexander Technique
142 West End Ave.
New York NY 10023
(212) 799-0468

Body awareness training. List of its members is available.

American Holistic Medical Association
6932 Little River Turnpike
Annandale VA 22003
(703) 642-5880

Referrals to holistic medical practioners.

American Massage & Therapy Association
Box 1270
Kingsport TN 37660
(615) 245-8071

Referrals to its members.

Association for Transpersonal Psychology
Box 3049
Stanford CA 94305
(415) 327-2066

Referrals to its member professionals.

Association of Holistic Health
Box 9352
San Diego CA 92109
(619) 275-2694

Directory of holistic health professionals.

Center for Traditional Acupuncture
Suite 108
American Cities Building
Columbia MD 21044
(301) 752-5425

Referrals to its trained practioners.

Dialogue House
80 East 11th St.
New York NY 10003
(212) 673-5880

Training in Journal Work and Dialoguing, as developed by Ira Progoff.

Eupsychia, Inc.
Box 3090
Austin TX 78764
(512) 327-2795

Training in Holotropic Breathwork (as developed by Stan and Christine Grof) with a particular slant toward healing addictions.

Feldenkrais Guild
Box 11145
San Francisco CA 94101
(415) 550-8708

List of Feldenkrais therapists.

HEAL
(Human Ecology Action League)
7330 North Rogers Ave.
Chicago IL 60626
(312) 665-6575

Information on environmental illness and physicians who specialize in it.

Hellerwork
147 Lomita Drive, Suite H
Mill Valley CA 94941
(415) 383-4240

List of trained practioners of its deep tissue bodywork. An off-shoot of Rolfing, Hellerwork places greater emphasis on body awareness and movement.

Integral Yoga Institue
227 West 13th St.
New York NY 10011
(212) 929-0586

Training in yoga and meditation. Branches throughout country.

LivingQuest
3962 Fuller Court
Boulder CO 80303
(303) 499-3440

Mail order books and tapes relating to eating disorders, health and transformation.

Price-Pottenger Nutrition Foundation
Box 2614
La Mesa CA 92041
(714) 582-4168

Publishes and sells an excellent selection of materials on nutrition.

Psychosynthesis International
Box 926
Diamond Springs CA 95619
(916) 622-9615

Information of psychosynthesis and the work of Edith Stauffer.

Rolf Institute
Box 1868
Boulder CO 80302
(303) 449-5903

Directory of trained practioners of its deep tissue bodywork.

SUGGESTED READING

No-Diet

Are you Hungry? A Completely New Approach to Raising Children Free of Food and Weight Problems by Jane R. Hirschmann and Lela Zaphiropoulos. Teach your child to trust his or her own hunger and satiety. Does away with concepts of "good" and "bad" foods. Exposes harmful attitudes.

The Dieter's Dilemma/Eating Less and Weighing More by William Bennett and Joel Gurin. Explains setpoint theory. Cites research. Proposes new attitude toward weight that accepts human diversity and recognizes many different styles of beauty.

Dieting Makes You Fat by Geoffrey Cannon and Hetty Einzig. The authors show how they freed themselves from the diet trap and found successful weight control through exercise and sound, whole nutrition.

*Don't Diet by Dale M. Atrens, Ph.D. Newest medical research exposes the myths of diets and fatness. The real facts prove that being overweight does not by itself make you unhealthy or unattractive. Nor does fatness cause heart disease, cancer or early death.

Stop Dieting, Start Living by Sharon Greene Patton. Excellent first-hand testimonial. Once a victim of the diet/binge syndrome, she tells how she became free to fight back and win. Exposes myths and fallacies of dieting.

Eating Disorders and Addictions

Anorexia Nervosa: Finding the Life Line by Patricia M. Stein and Barbara C. Unell. Recovering anorexics tell their own stories. This book is good for anyone from junior high age and up.

Breaking Free from Compulsive Eating by Geneen Roth. Geneen's experience with her own problems of overeating combined with the experience gathered from her "Breaking Free" workshops makes this an informative and practical guide.

Compulsive Overeater by Bill B. Bill's personal testimonial on the twelve steps of the Overeaters Anonymous program.

Coping with Bulimia by Barbara French. A refreshingly simple account describing Bulimia — what it is, how it differs from Anorexia and how it can be tackled and defeated.

Diets Don't Work by Bob Schwartz. A step-by-step guide in workbook format designed to help you discover why you are overweight and how to take the weight off without dieting. Emphasis is on developing a new self-image based on being a naturally thin person. Exercises for self-awareness and change.

Fat is a Family Affair by Judi Hollis. This is one of the few books I've seen that talks to the family member of the compulsive overeater, as well as to the compulsive eater, about your special relationship and what you both have to do to change for recovery.

Fat is a Feminist Issue and *Fat is a Feminist Issue II*, both by Susie Orbach. Exercises to help you discover what purpose bingeing and overweight have in your life and how to change.

Feeding the Hungry Heart by Geneen Roth. Stories direct from the hearts of those who suffer from overweight and compulsive eating. A very moving book. Offers hope and inspiration.

The Hungry Self by Kim Chernin. Explores the often troubled relationship between mothers and daughters. Shows how daughters use an obsession with food to flee the struggle for identity and self-development.

The Journey Within: A Spiritual Path to Recovery by Ruth Fishel. This recovering alcoholic leads you through affirmations, visualizations and meditations along the spiritual path to recovery.

Making Peace with Food by Susan Kano. Step-by-step guide. Relearn the basics behind natural weight control. Understand why you are troubled and how to break free. Learn how to estimate your setpoint, listen to and love your body, eat spontaneously and express your needs. Emphasis is on freeing yourself from an obsessive food mentality.

Maintenance for Compulsive Overeaters: The Twelve Step Way to Ongoing Recovery by Bill B. Valuable insights about achieving and maintaining a healthy, lasting recovery from compulsive overeating by the author of *Compulsive Overeater*. Highlighted by nineteen personal stories of recovery.

The Monster Within by Cynthia Joye Rowland. A first-hand account of Cynthia's struggle with bulimia and her painful battle for recovery. Insights into the causes of her illness would be of value to anyone grappling with this insidious disease.

My Name is Caroline by Caroline Adams Miller. Caroline Miller's story of her battle with bulimia and her involvement with a self-help fellowship.

The Obsession by Kim Chernin. A beautifully written analysis of our society's demand that women be thin. A thought-provoking discussion as to the reasons men have encouraged this obsession and women have embraced it.

Stage II Recovery by Earnie Larson. Based on the premise that the result of all addiction is low self-esteem (and therefore, our inability to have satisfying relationships) he has devised a simple (not to be mistaken with easy) program to help understand and change the underlying living problems that cause unhappiness.

Stage II Relationships by Earnie Larson. Making relationships work is at the heart of full recovery from addictions. This book explores this theme in depth, offering sound advice and practical techniques for breaking unhealthy patterns of behavior that linger after abstinence has been achieved.

Starving for Attention by Cherry Boone O'Neill. Cherry's moving and inspirational account of her struggle with Anorexia Nervosa and recovery.

Such a Pretty Face by Marcia Millman. Through case studies, personal testimonials and by observing such organizations as the National Association to Aid Fat Americans, Overeaters Anonymous and a children's diet camp, we are given insight into the political and social realm, as well as the experience of being fat in America.

Weight Loss from the Inside Out by Marion Bilich. In order to lose weight and keep it off you must first discover what purpose fat has in your life. This book will help you do just that.

*When Society Becomes an Addict by Anne Wilson Schaef. Identifies addiction as the underlying malaise of our culture. Through a remarkable synthesis of feminist, chemical dependency and mental health theories, Schaef introduces the addictive process, explores its attributes and points the way to functioning outside the system. It is a powerful and convincing argument for abandoning a system in which self-centeredness, dishonesty, the illusion of control and constant crises are the norm.

Body Awareness

The Body Book by David Bodanis. A wonderful job of illustrating the most intricate workings of our inner cosmos. What happens when we are angry, fearful, worried, sick, relaxed or experience pain? The drama taking place at the molecular level is at least as exciting as your favorite soap opera. The narrative is intriguing, sometimes even humorous, and the photos are beautiful.

The Book of Massage by Lucinda Lidell. One of the best on the subject. Beautifully illustrated, it is a clear and concise step-by-step guide to the techniques of massage, shiatsu and reflexology.

I Love My Body by Louise L. Hay. A 30-day affirmation guide designed to help you create a new, beautiful, healthier and happier body. There are affirmations for 30 parts of the body — hips, stomach, waistline, mouth, mind, etc. If you are having trouble seeing the beauty in your body parts, this book could be a big help.

New Our Bodies, Ourselves by The Boston Women's Health Book Collective. A classic book for women on all aspects of women's health —one of the most complete sourcebooks on women's health care issues available to date. This book is especially important for the women who have been brainwashed by the media's stereotyping of women's roles and looks. The perspectives given will help release the power and energy that has been trapped by attitudes and conditions which restrict thinking, not only about weight and body image, but also about the total functioning of our bodies as women and as people.

Relaxed Body Book by the Editors of American Health Magazine with Daniel Goleman, Ph.D. and Tara Bennett-Goleman. Release stress that has accumulated in your body through a variety of techniques: massage, acupressure, yoga, Alexander and Feldenkrais. These exercises will help you feel great.

The Sivananda Companion to Yoga by The Sivananda Yoga Center. A classic guide to hatha yoga — very clear, comprehensive and superbly illustrated. Yoga has been a vehicle for people transforming the quality of their lives for thousands of years.

Stretching by Bob Anderson. Stretching relaxes the mind and tunes the body. America's leading stretching expert teaches you how to stretch the right way. There are stretches for every part of your body, special stretching routines for specific sports, exercises for developing strength, special techniques for running and cycling and a chapter on caring for your back.

The Teenage Body Book by Kathey McCoy and Charles Wibbelsman, M.D. Everything the teenager wants to know about his/her body. Some topics include: woman's body, man's body, changing feelings, dangers of dieting, overweight, eating disorders, exercise and sports, stress, changing habit patterns, sexuality, birth control, pregnancy, sexually transmitted diseases and where to go for help.

*Transforming Body Image by Marcia Germaine Hutchinson. The only book of its kind that I know of. An invaluable source of exercises designed to help you transform a negative body image into a positive one. A must!

Personal Growth/Self-Help

*At a Journal Workshop by Ira Progoff. Dr. Progoff has developed a unique method of journal writing. The Intensive Journal process is a series of progressive exercises (daily log, twilight imagery, time-stretch-

ing, dialoguing, and more) which will help you reconnect with the inner content and continuity of your life. An exceptional method.

Celebrate Your Self by Dorothy Corville Briggs. Becoming aware of our past programming is the first step to freedom. Commitment to change is the second. Briggs will show you how in this highly inspirational and instructive book. Learn the difference between your "self-image" and the Real You.

*Creative Visualization by Shakti Gawain. Gives meditations, exercises and techniques that can become part of your everyday routine to create the things you want and increase your personal mastery of life.

*The Creative Visualization Workbook by Shakti Gawain. The companion to *Creative Visualization*. Learn to set goals, clear out negative belief systems and connect with your creativity and intuition.

*Dr. Weisinger's Anger Work-Out Book by Hendrie Weisinger, Ph.D. A workbook designed to help you find constructive ways of dealing with anger. Good for those who, although they don't experience anger directly, feel the painful effects of repressed anger, including low self-esteem, depression and substance abuse.

Feeling Good by David D. Burns, M.D. A cognitive therapeutic approach to dealing with emotions.

From Fear to Freedom by Darlene Deer Truchses. Will provide insight and understanding as to how women's self-esteem has been affected by the very roles we've been expected to play in society. The author, through her own personal quest, brings deep insight into the specific problems that many women face: "how to combine self-actualization or personal power with. . . the nurturing, caring, loving and accepting characteristics that are so valuable" and are already so much a part of the female spirit.

*Giving Away Success by Susan Schenkel. Speaks to all women. Explains why lack of confidence, feelings of helplessness, fear of failure and lack of assertiveness affect our ability to succeed. I saw myself in every page. Tools for getting "unstuck." If you are female, and if you have trouble going to where you want to go, I highly recommend this book.

Inner Work by Robert A. Johnson. In-depth instruction on how to work with dreams and "active imagination."

Living in the Light by Shakti Gawain. Valuable information on what intuition is and how to use it; how to become "a creative channel;" how to keep our commitment to our higher selves and still enjoy all the worldly things around us.

Positive Addiction by William Glasser, M.D. Gain strength and self-esteem by replacing negative addictions (such as overeating) with positive ones (such as jogging, meditation, etc.). A thought provoking and inspiring book.

Unlimited Power by Anthony Robbins. A highly accessible and entertaining introduction to neuro-linguistic programming. NLP offers some valuable techniques for changing ourselves and our relationships.

Visualization: Directing the Movies of Your Mind by Adelaide Bry. Will show you how to use visualization to improve your life: create the life you want for yourself, improve health, replay the movies of your childhood, expand your mind to improve creativity.

Why Me? Garrett Porter & Patricia A. Norris, Ph.D. This 9-year old boy healed himself of a terminal brain tumor through the use of visualization. The story of his recovery in his own words combined with Dr. Norris' explanation of how to work with visualization for healing makes this a truly remarkable book.

You Can Heal Your Life by Louise L. Hay. Heal yourself through positive affirmation — release resentments and practice forgiveness. Louise will show you how.

Unconditional Love and Forgiveness by Edith R. Stauffer. An unusual and very interesting book, based on two bodies of work: the ancient Essene Code of Conduct and psychosynthesis, a holistic, transpersonal psychology created by Roberto Assagioli, M.D. This unique process of forgiveness has been found "to be immensely beneficial for those desiring to free themselves of hostility and resentment."

Audio Listening

Loving Yourself with Louise Hay. A beautiful and inspirational combination of music and songs by Jai Josephs and meditations by Louise Hay. Joyous celebration of ourselves. Songs lift the heart; meditations help reprogram subconscious programming.

Morning & Evening Meditations with Louise Hay. Open each day with thankfulness and positive affirmation for what the day will bring. Close each day with gratitude for all that has been experienced and prepare yourself for deep and restful sleep.

Healing the Inner Child with Jacquelyn Small. A beautiful guided exercise which has much potential for healing. Excellent for anyone dealing with addictions.

Vipassana Meditation with Jacquelyn Small. A simple meditation technique clearly explained. Excellent for the beginning meditator.

---

* Can be ordered from LivingQuest, 3962-B Fuller Ct., Boulder CO 80303. Send for free catalog.

INDEX